Primary Health Care: A Global Outlook

Primary Health Care: A Global Outlook

Edited by **Kelly Ward**

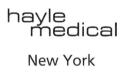

hayle medical

New York

Published by Hayle Medical,
30 West, 37th Street, Suite 612,
New York, NY 10018, USA
www.haylemedical.com

Primary Health Care: A Global Outlook
Edited by Kelly Ward

International Standard Book Number: 978-1-63241-325-3 (Hardback)

Printed in the United States of America.

Contents

Preface

The purpose of the book is to provide a glimpse into the dynamics and to present opinions and studies of some of the scientists engaged in the development of new ideas in the field from very different standpoints. This book will prove useful to students and researchers owing to its high content quality.

"In both, clinical practitioners and scientists, few find it more convenient to depend upon irrelevant clarifications, while the rest never stop looking for answers". With these astonishing words, Augusto Murri, an Italian veteran in clinical medicine, emphasizes on the fact that medical practice must be a constant journey towards knowledge and quality of care. This book is a compilation of contributions from across the globe. Distinct cultures are portrayed together, from those with developed technologies to those of indefinite spirituality, but they are all associated to each other through 5 professional characteristics, that in the 1978 the Institute of Medicine (IOM) stated as most important for practicing good Primary Care: coordination, accessibility, accountability, comprehensiveness and continuity. The content in this book is organized under three characteristics - accountability, comprehensiveness and continuity. An international overview of hot topics and novel insights will be available to the readers.

At the end, I would like to appreciate all the efforts made by the authors in completing their chapters professionally. I express my deepest gratitude to all of them for contributing to this book by sharing their valuable works. A special thanks to my family and friends for their constant support in this journey.

Editor

Section 1

Accessibility to Primary Care

Public Health in Primary Care

L. Cegolon[1,2], G. Mastrangelo[2] and J. H. Lange[3]
[1]Padua University, Department of Molecular Medicine, Padua,
[2]Imperial College London, School of Public Health, S. Mary's Campus, London,
[3]Envirosafe Training and Consultants, Pittsburgh, Pennsylvania,
[1]Italy
[2]UK
[3]USA

1. Introduction

"*Primary health care*' is a political concept widely defined as "*the mobilization of various forces in society (health professionals, institutions, lay people) around an agenda of transformation of health systems that is driven by the social values of equity, solidarity and participation*"; "*primary care*" instead refers more specifically to technical aspects of the Care and services delivered by the health system, more toward evidence-based medicine [van Weel 2012, WHO 2008b, Kruk 2010].

Good primary care foundations furnish a number of benefits to a health system: better health for the population served, broad and equitable access to services, preparedness, an appropriate approach for disease prevention, and financial protection [Piterman 2005, WHO 2000]. Peculiarities of primary care are in fact first-contact care, ease of access, care for a broad range of health needs, continuity, and involvement of the family and community ["Declaration of Alma-Ata" 1978, Kekki 2006, Starfield 1992, van Well 2012, Kruk 2010].

Primary care systems have been frequently compared to secondary care-centered systems [Atun 2004, Engstrom 2001, Health Council of the Netherlands 2004, Macinko 2003, Starfield 2005]. Well organized primary care systems seem better able to tackle the new challenges of modern societies and the changing pattern of disease than hospital-oriented health care [WHO 2008a/b]. Furthermore, by guiding patients through the system, primary care physicians (PCP) become a key element to better address and respond to the needs of patients along with an understanding of a patient's concerns with their health and care, which in many ways is patient centered care [van Weel, 2012, Schafer 2011]. Indeed primary care enables access to care for the general population as well as for specific groups [Uiters 2009].

Moreover the implementation of some primary care measures (e.g. having a primary care physician as a regular health care provider, the availability of community health centers focusing on primary care, etc.) was found to be beneficial in terms of health outcomes [Franks 1998, Starfield 1992, Starfield 2005, Villalbi 1999, Kruk 2010].

A national health system founded on primary care can therefore theoretically improve the possibilities of performance because:

- primary (unlike secondary) care plays an integrative role;
- health care is more accessible;
- it reinforces the relationship between primary and secondary care;
- care is better appropriated, as based on an evidence based approach;
- all health care resources are organized and rationalized by targeting the promotion, maintenance, and improvement of health.

2. Primary care and public health

Primary care and public health medicine originated in the nineteenth century, with PCPs evolving as separate clinical specialists; although, this emergence had commonalities [Piterman 2005]. This broad area of medicine developed in response to issues of urbanization, as a result of the changing needs of the community, the birth/expansion of epidemiology and integration of evidence-based medicine [van Well 2012, Hannay 1993].

However physicians with strict clinical responsibilities and lacking formal public health training did not have the management background required for public health positions. Public health medicine was responsible to set targets, allocate resources, evaluate progress, control communicable diseases, and promote health. Public health specialists were the main source of medical advice for health authorities.

Preventive services, which most commonly include, but are not limited to, immunization, health promotion, disease prevention and family planning, were initially assigned to medical officers responsible for health in Great Britain in 1919. However , service fees being collected by PCPs to provide this preventive care at the same time were encouraged as well [BMA 1993, Hannay 1993].

Primary care and public health medicine have been pursuing different paths, with PCPs having little epidemiology training and public health doctors hardly noting how PCPs were becoming more formally responsible for promoting health and preventing disease in Great Britain [UK Faculty of Public Health 1992].

The relevance of primary care in modern health systems can be perceived by the budget recently allocated by the British government into the Primary Care Trusts (PCT), the centre of the UK National Health System (NHS) responsible for spending around 75-80% of the total NHS budget [NHS 2010].

The paths of primary care and public health medicine have recently come closer: epidemiology was given credibility by clinical contact, and PCPs were made responsible for health promotion and disease prevention for the first time at the end of last century in Great Britain [Morrell 1991]. In the attempt to further attenuate these barriers postgraduate master's courses became available to PCPs and public health physicians were appointed managers at primary care services [Hannay 1993]. Nowadays both PCPs and public health doctors are responsible for preventing disease and promoting health. PCPs deal not only with the clinical management of the general community, but they also serve as front line public health officers. Today PCPs need to work within the broader context of "*primary health care*", requiring approach of medical care for individual patients combined with health promotion of populations [Hannay 1993]. Also, the integration of primary care and public health is important for tackling health inequalities, especially in areas with low social cohesion.

3. Preventive medicine and health promotion in primary care

As cost containment occurred in health care today there has been a shift from curative toward preventive medicine, with the aim of keeping and maintaining health rather than waiting until illness occurs to treat the patient.

Preventive care's main focus is on diseases prevention, which also requires skills in populations and community medicine beside clinical medicine. However, as they see the individual rather than the population many PCPs do not receive proper training in preventative medicine.

Albeit the ultimate target is the individual, either public health services or primary care clinical facilities could take responsibility for organizing primary prevention programs (e.g. health education or immunization campaigns), secondary prevention programs (e.g. screening or targeted health education) and tertiary prevention programs (e.g. health surveys to document unmet needs) [Starfield 1996].

3.1 Non communicable diseases

Beside the positive aspect that most people nowadays live longer, the ageing population in developed countries is generating a number of relevant consequences: health issues have today shifted from acute/communicable diseases to chronic and long-term conditions, as well as being lifestyle related [Schafer 2011]. Non-communicable diseases (NCD) represent a significant and unfortunately growing burden worldwide. Chronic conditions as neuropsychiatric disorders, cardiovascular disease and cancer account for most of the burden of disease [WHO 2008c]. In the past NCD mainly afflicted developed countries, but nowadays they have become a major health problem in the developing world too and will become even more widespread. Developing countries are indeed shifting towards a western lifestyle of unhealthy diet and physical inactivity and this will enhance the rate of NCDs [Wagner 2011, Lam 2012, Hu 2011]. Although some conditions do not cause death, it is important to take non-fatal conditions into account, when assessing the causes of loss of health in populations and the disability-adjusted life-years (DALYs) lost [WHO 2012a]. These factors are critical in enhancing the quality of life. Moreover it is important to note that chronic disorders appear to be correlated with each other, as suggested for cardiovascular diseases (CVDs) and neuropsychiatric conditions [Preisig 2011].

For the prevention and management of chronic conditions there is evidence that primary care is more cost-effective as compared to secondary care [Baicker 2004, Franks 1998; Welch 1993]. The integration of primary care, social care and family context of patients is an ideal approach to support people in self-managing their long-term conditions and to facilitate their living longer at home and in the community [Boerma 1998, Gress 2009].

CVD prevention is a good example in illustrating how primary care could be effective in disease prevention.

Risk factors for CVDs are established; although, some of them are not modifiable (namely age, sex, genetics), for others much can be done in terms of health promotion to eliminate/attenuate the underlying risk [Mitchell 2010]. Smoking, poor diet and lack of physical activity are indeed the main causes for CVDs. The consequences of an unhealthy life style are well known: overweight; unbalanced ratio total cholesterol/HDL and elevated blood pressure [Katzmarzyk 2004].

Reduction of CVD risk can be effectively accomplished by smoking cessation, a reduced intake of saturated fatty acids (that will ultimately decrease the level of LDL and total cholesterol), a reduced salt intake (beneficial for hypertension) and consuming fruits, vegetables and foods rich in fibers and micronutrients that can be protective against CVDs. An hypo-caloric diet along with physical activity are also protective against obesity and may result in improvement of the cardiovascular system [Britton 2011]. Primary care is an ideal setting to efficiently deliver health education programs aiming to target all the above preventive measures, thanks to the continuous, privileged and long-running clinical contact of PCPs with their patients. One of the problems today has been to prescribe statins as a substitute, from a practical prospective, rather than addressing the underlining causes (e.g. obesity).

Drinking (alcohol) education and smoking cessation are reportedly difficult tasks to achieve. Despite numerous advances in tobacco-dependence treatment, U.S. adult smoking prevalence and quit rates have indeed stalled [Abrams 2007, Orleans 2007, Gollbust 2008]. According to Levy [2010] the annual smoking cessation without any intervention is estimated as being 4.3%, reaching a rate of 4.5-10% with corporate health education campaigns requiring great effort and resources. Furthermore relapse rates after cessation are reported to be as high as cessation according to Hughes [2008], Hajek [2009] and Anderson [2009]. Yet efforts to prevent teens from taking up smoking have shown no evidence of long-term effectiveness [Wiehe 2005]. This is also seen for some occupational groups (e.g. asbestos abatement workers) where there has been no change in smoking rates over the last 20 years despite strong and repeated warnings and education [Lange 2011].

Furthermore prevalence of binge and heavy drinking among adults in the United States has been practically constant from 1993–2009, with approximately 5% of the total population drinking heavily, while 15% of the population binge drink [Centers for Disease Control and Prevention - CDC 2012]. According to a review conducted by Foxcroft [2003] about the effectiveness of short- and medium-term primary intervention for alcohol misuse in young people, no firm conclusions have proven to be possible. Health education campaigns have failed to achieve significant public health results over time in reducing alcohol misuse.

New corporate strategies should therefore be planned to tackle smoking and alcohol misuse, combining health education campaigns involving different key figures (PCPs, pharmacists, the media, school teachers, counselors) with Government measures such as sales regulation and taxation. Moreover recent recommendations from the WHO indicate workplace health promotion as a pre-requisite for sustainable social and economic development for nations as a strategy for prevention [WHO 2012b]. As people spend more time at work today it is also important to involve occupational physicians in these multi-agency teams aiming at health promotion.

The workplace is in fact an environment where:

- a substantial percentage of the general population accrues;
- informal leaders and officials are delegated to promote health and safety at work;
- individuals (workers) are more receptive to health education.

Hence the workplace health promotion would enable to reach all of those individuals with difficulties in seeing their PCPs during their working hours. However PCPs remain essential figures to deal with the rest of the population, especially elderly and children.

Although not mentioned in the WHO Comparative Risk Assessment (CRA) module of the Global Burden of Disease [Ezzati 2002, The Lancet 2011], the ethnical background [Cruz-Flores 2011] and the educational level and socio-economic status [Agardh 2011] of patients appear to be correlated with chronic conditions or influencing other risk factors as smoking [Harris 2011] or obesity [Seidell 1997]. Health education should therefore cautiously be planned considering these variables.

Another aspect that cannot be ignored by PCPs is being a "good example" for their patients in terms of health behavior. It has in fact been shown that endorsement of physical activity is more credible coming from a health professional that also practices physical activity. PCPs should practice physical activity themselves, not only for their own benefit, but also as a stimulus for their patients [Abramson 2000, Orrow 2012]. The same concept applies to smoking, drinking and diet.

Despite the need of further improvement, mortality for CVDs and in some ways diabetes in various Western countries has reached overall good results [WHO 2011, Reaven 2011, Rosamond 2012], thanks to the health care resources allocated and the public health campaigns deployed over the past years. By contrast, in many developing countries type II diabetes is growing at epidemic levels [Hu 2011, Lam 2012]. Overall, prevention of type II diabetes through health education aiming at moderate diet and lifestyle modifications should be a primary function of PCPs and falls in the basic domain of public health [Schulze 2011].

Furthermore in Eastern European countries that have attempted to transform and up-date their healthcare systems over the past two decades, just after the fall of communism, CVDs still account for the vast majority of deaths in these areas [WHO Europe 2004, WHO 2011].

Since the 1990s, policy makers in Central and Eastern Europe have supported reforms leading towards primary care [Windak 2005]. Also in other countries of Europe, such as Spain, Greece and Portugal, reforms of health systems have aimed to strengthen primary care [Campbell 2005]. There is now a strong need for evidence to monitor and support these developments in Europe.

Integrated approaches have been proposed focusing on the main common risk factors for a range of chronic conditions: CVDs, diabetes and cancer: unhealthy diet, physically inactivity and tobacco use [WHO 2012b].

However, the health achievements obtained for CVDs and diabetes have not been met in cancer prevention. In fact malignancies are becoming the leading cause of death in high-income countries. The crossover of cancer to heart disease mortality has indeed been recently reported in US [US National Center for Health Statistics 2006], New Zealand [New Zealand Information Service 2003], France [WHO Europe 2004,WHO Global infobase] Spain [WHO Europe 2004], Canada [Statistics Canada 2009] and Netherlands [Statistics Netherland 2008]. These figures highly suggest failing outcomes in cancer prevention combined with rather effective measures to tackle and prevent CVDs. However, environmental pollution may also be playing a factor in a lack of change or even increase for cancer rates.

As of behavioral risk, previous observational studies showed that cancer could be prevented by a high intake of fruits and vegetables; however the European Prospective Investigation into Cancer and Nutrition cohort (EPIC, 142,605 men and 335,873 women) provided evidence of a very small inverse association between fruit and vegetable intake and cancer risk [Boffetta 2010]. Likewise, in two prospective cohorts (71,910 women in the Nurses' Health study and 37,725 men in the Health Professionals' Follow-up Study) healthy eating based on a fruit and vegetable diet proved to be effective in reducing CVDs but not cancer incidence [Hung 2004]. Furthermore, as mentioned above, satisfying and long lasting results in the reduction of alcoholism and smoking cessation are hard to reach. Ex-smokers also continue to have an elevated risk of developing lung cancer for a number of years after smoking cessation [Anthonisen 2005, Ebbert 2003], probably as a result of absence of further insult on epithelial cells rather than reversal of existing disease or genetic changes [Anthonisen 2005].

Despite all this evidence, the Union for International Cancer Control (UICC) still suggested in 2005 the same key risk factors for cancer prevention: tobacco and alcohol consumption, weight/high BMI, sun exposure, and infections [UICC 2005].

Apart from trying to improve the current public health strategies against drinking and smoking, new research should be devoted towards innovative approaches for cancer prevention (e.g. chemo-prophylaxis [Hobhom 2009]) that could be applied in more effective anti-cancer health promotion campaigns.

3.2 Communicable diseases

Initial cases of infectious disease are usual seen at the primary care level [Hogg 2006, Glasgow 2008]. This makes the PCPs an important sentinel in disease identification and reporting. Without a good understanding of infectious disease and epidemiology, such events can be easily missed. This requires the PCP to be an investigator of infectious diseases most often without a full picture of the actual event. Such diseases have been recently shown to impact the health care industry, especially for those events involving highly infectious agents such as influenza [Winchester, 2009], tuberculosis [Sablan 2009] or Severe Acute Respiratory Syndrome (SARS) [Lange 2005]. Early detection can mitigate a disease's spread and reduce the potential of an epidemic [Wong 2005]. Although such event is uncommon on a regional or global scale, outbreaks commonly occur at the local level [Lau 2010]. Primary care can provide an invaluable contribution for the Initial identification of an outbreak.

For example, this can be seen for occurrence of pertussis (*Bordetella pertussis*). Today, even many of the diseases considered to be associated with childhood are now occurring in adults (e.g. pertussis) [CDC 2003]. Here such events are generally related to a lack of preventative practice, in this case failure to adequately vaccinate or failing in determining the current status of vaccination level. This can even be extended to the occupational environment where a pertussis outbreak occurred in a group of oil refinery workers [CDC 2003].

In most cases, outbreaks at the local level are most commonly associated with food poisoning. In locations where reporting is mandatory, it has been found that actual notification is poor with a trend even declining [Day 2007]. Such practices do not allow the full realization of disease rate and can perpetuate an endemic event. This becomes even more important with the finding that there are 200 cases of gastrointestinal disease for every 1,000 registered patients a year in England [Day 2007]. However, the delay in laboratory reporting sometimes can be considerable. For example, in Australia there is a 19 day delay for *Bordetella pertussis* and many PCPs have a poor understanding of the time line and process, especially on its impact for controlling a communicable disease [Allen 2000]. As a result the spread of a disease can be magnified, especially one that is high communicable, as influenza [Khan 2012]. Information and reports from PCPs are key components in establishing disease registrations and surveillance along with describing events for estimating future trends [Day 2007]. As mentioned, these preventative activities apply not only to patients but those in occupations that are at risk (e.g. health-care workers, industrial populations). A lack of preventative measures at the occupational level can allow a local event (epidemic) to occur. PCPs can be effective in preventing infectious disease through health education, by informing patients on preventative practices. One of the key domains in this regard is vaccination against traditional diseases such as tetanus toxoid, hepatitis B, mumps, measles, rubella, diphtheria, polio, meningitis, Haemophilus influenza, pneumococcus, yellow fever and (more recently) varicella [Bilcke 2012]. Proper vaccination, especially against continuing and emerging-related diseases remains an important area for PCPs, frequently forgotten with consideration given to more high technology activities [Venkat 2012]. Evaluation as to whether a patient's vaccine schedule is up-to-date is a fundamental practice in primary care.

Another important mechanism to reduce the transmission of various infectious diseases is hand-washing [Bencho 2006].

4. Environmental and occupational medicine

Occupational diseases (e.g. particulate induced asthma) are major hazards which can mostly be prevented [Rosenblatt 2005]. Since they are most likely to be the first to encounter patients with these types of problems [Weevers 2005], PCPs are in many ways gatekeepers in recognizing and in some ways preventing environmental and occupational diseases. However, as their focus is on clinical identification and treatment of the disease, PCPs are normally not trained to recognize occupational diseases. In environmental and occupational medicine the critical point is not a clinical diagnosis of the disease, but rather the etiological diagnosis (e.g. agent of causation) [Cegolon 2010b]. The answer to four easy questions in occupational medicine history taking is helpful for an initial assessment of the possible disease causation [Agius 2000, Cegolon 2010b]:

-   *Temporal relationship*: What is the time lag between the initial exposure and the start of the symptoms ?
-   *Dose-effect (time) relationship*: do the symptoms improve if the patient is not exposed any longer (e.g. if he/she changes work duties or is on holiday)?
-   *Dose-effect relationship*: do the symptoms worsen if the patient carries out specific duties or works in areas characterised by high levels of exposure?
-   *Strength of the association*: are colleagues affected by the same symptoms related to the same exposure?

As environmental pollution and the number of chemicals/agents in the occupational environment increase, it can be hard to establish a relationship between a disease and a specific agent. This can be magnified when interactions among different exposure agents are considered. Identification of this nature is often required by regulatory and insurance agencies for compensation and future prevention [Liss 2011]. Initial assessment may be possible by the type of personal protective equipment (PPE) used by the patient; in fact there are different forms of PPE and each has varying value in providing protection against harmful agents [Health and Safety Executive -HSE 1999, Garrod 2003, Agius 2000, La Dou 2008]. Much of this can be accomplished through obtaining an adequate medical history.

Most of these diseases are duration related; therefore, a history of time and concentration exposure is required to suspect an environmental and occupational disease/diagnosis. Nevertheless, recognition and understanding the causation of occupational diseases is critical, as the latency period often makes it difficult to assess the exposure.

What is of even greater importance is the prevention of future disease cases in the population and origin of the patient. This practice is only slightly within the realm of primary care. However, PCPs are an important resource to alert others more directly responsible for preventing such occurrences.

This also requires an understanding of changes in recognizable diseases related to the work environment, as the case of asbestos in the western world. Historically, asbestos has been considered a contributor to occupational respiratory disease. However, due to controls and better understanding of this mineral agent, those engaging in its abatement (asbestos abatement workers) have low exposure and little or even no risk of developing disease directly as a result of this agent [Lange 2011]. What have become of importance in disease causation for this occupational population are confounders such as their personal habits (e.g. smoking) and risk characteristics, aspects so far mostly ignored with focus on actual asbestos exposure. These concepts are continually changing and require PCPs to keep up-to-date their current knowledge in the areas they practice. PCPs must therefore assess the actual disease risk through evidence-based medicine.

5. Global health

It has been estimated that environmental causes account for about 25% of global related diseases [Gehle 2011]. Global warming and an increased level of pollutants on a world-wide basis are changing the biometric characteristics and the environment in various geographical locations in an unpredicted manner. Change in the global environment has therefore brought about a difference in diseases seen in primary care. For example increased heat stress and related events not normally seen in different areas are now emerging [Hajat 2010]. Depletion of the stratospheric ozone layer has led to increased solar UV-B radiation at the surface of the earth leading to increased human exposure to UV-B radiation with consequent detrimental and beneficial effects on health, most notably on the eye (cataract) and the skin (cancer) [Norval 2011]. A rise in infectious disease rates will also be likely impacted by global and regional warming/pollution [Semenza 2011]. Furthermore, the extent and severity of asthma is increasing, requiring a larger number of visits and more aggressive treatments [Rosenblatt 2005]. This change in rate and severity cannot be offset by immunization and may even be magnified by changing patterns of influenza and other infectious diseases. These new scenarios will increase the primary care workload, as these conditions will be handled in many ways by PCPs. Many of the culprits of this climate changes are beyond controls of medicine, but the outcomes will have to be dealt with by those at the front line.

As populations increase, primary care will grow in importance, as for some it may become the only form of care accessible. Furthermore primary care will also likely change its role, as may need their PCPs to acquire additional sub-specialization.

For instance the health effects of hot weather are quickly becoming a global public health challenge of this century [Hajat 2010]. As heat related diseases are largely avoidable, various public health protection measures have been put in place in some cities across the world, with particular emphasis on preventive strategies for susceptible individuals [Keatinge 2003]. In particular it is fundamental for physicians and pharmacists to be prepared for effective prevention, first-aid treatment and knowledge of possible adverse effects of medicines prescribed during hot weather [Hajat 2010].

Overall, PCPs in the future will have to include a more comprehensive (global) approach in the management and diagnosis of diseases, as in some cases a condition is unrelated to the actual individual but their environment. The old approach treating a condition without a holistic view not considering possible underlying causes seems to be obsolete.

6. Research in primary care

Research in primary care is becoming more relevant, as it offers the opportunity to examine huge samples, more representative of the general population. PCP networks in many countries allow collection of large national electronic databases to be employed for several purposes: academic primary care research; disease monitoring; population's needs assessment; tracking changes over time (trends) and in response to interventions; pharmacological-vigilance; health care evaluation; infectious disease surveillance; outbreak investigation; clinical trials; etc [Medicine and Health Care Products Regulatory Agency - MHRA]. Most electronic health databases are used in pharmaco-epidemiologic studies [Schneeweiss 2005]. The General Practitioners Research Database (GPRD) for instance is an international electronic medical record system including basic demographic details, medical records, drug history, and prevention records. In addition to its comprehensive contents, linkages to external registries (e.g. Cancer Registry or Hospital Episodes Statistics database) are also made possible by sophisticated encryption procedures [Majeed 2004]. Access barriers to these national electronic databases should be reduced in order to make more data available for research. These data have great potential as research tools and can help in maximizing the outputs: in particular academic research and health care de;ivery [Chun Chen 2011]

Primary care research allows a more pragmatic approach than conventional randomized control trials (RCT, often funded by pharmaceutical companies and based at tertiary centres), as it provides a more realistic assessment of drug use and reflects a shared decision between PCPs and their respective patients. Patients' experiences with drugs in "real world" clinical practices are indeed particularly relevant. Furthermore primary care doctors rely on clinical judgment and experience to weigh the risks and benefits of trials [David 2008].

7. Primary care in prospects

Despite primary care aims at equity in the access and distribution of health services [Wilkinson 1990], recent research suggested that PCPs treating wealthier and more educated patients may be better trained clinically and may have more access to important clinical resources than physicians treating less affluent patients. Further research should be conducted to address the extent to which these differences may be responsible for disparities in health care [Bach 2004].

In western societies we are assisting a progressive individualization, with citizens becoming more autonomous in their decisions and less dependent and linked to their social environment [Mills 2007]. These societal developments are bringing people to stay more at home and being independent, but are also weakening social relations and cohesions [Schafer 2011].

Patients nowadays are more knowledgeable about medicine, demanding a higher standard of care and willing to get involved into health care decision making. More information is indeed nowadays available, especially through the internet [Groenewengen 2008, Schafer 2011].

The increasing relevance of markets in health care is having an impact on the competition at work, with health care workers expressing less trust in their colleagues and as a result generating a more fragmented work environment [Groenewengen 2008]. This is not helpful for the management, for instance, of chronic and long term conditions where integration and cooperation between the various health care providers involved is recommended. Cooperation, good relationships between primary and secondary care and integration of care between organizations are more important than competition [Schafer 2011].

There is considerable variation in the organization of primary care across Europe. Albeit this is positive as countries can learn from each other, there is also a need for a European infrastructure to support training and integrate primary care action. For instance some European countries are still lacking academic primary care programs and academic institutions, invaluable instruments to monitor health outcomes and evaluate health systems [De Maeseneer 2010].

Modern primary care needs to evolve from a family business into a larger, corporate organization, both at the national and international level [Schafer 2011].

8. References

Ab Rahman A, Ab Rahman R, Ibrahim MI, et al. Knowledge of sexual and reproductive health among adolescents attending school in Kelantan, Malaysia. Southeast Asian J Trop Med Public Health. 2011;42:717-25.

Abrams D. Comprehensive smoking cessation policy for all smokers: systems integration to save lives and money. In: Bonnie RJ, Stratton K, Wallace RB, eds. Ending the tobacco problem: a blueprint for the nation. Washington: The National Academies Press. 2007.

Abramson S, Stein J, Schaufele M, Frates E, Rogan S. Personal exercise habits and counseling practices of primary care physicians: a national survey. Clin J Sport Med. 2000;10:40-8.

Agardh EE et al. Burden of type 2 diabetes attributed to lower educational levels in Sweden. Population Health Metrics. 2011, 9:60.

Agius R: Taking an Occupational History. Health Environment & Work 2000 [http://www.agius.com/hew/resource/occhist.htm]. (updated in January 2010; accessed on 23 July 2011).

Allen CJ, Ferson MJ. Notification of infectious diseases by general practitioners: a quantitative and qualitative study. Med J Aust. 2000;172:325-8.

Anderson CM, Yip R, Henschke CI, Yankelevitz DF, Ostroff JS, Burns DM. Smoking Cessation and Relapse during a Lung Cancer Screening Program. Cancer Epidemiol Biomarkers Prev. 2009;18: 3476-83.

Anthonisen NR, Skeans MA, Wise RA, Manfreda J, Kanner RE, Connett JE .The Effects of a Smoking Cessation Intervention on 14.5-Year Mortality. Ann Intern Med. 2005;142: 233-239.

Atun, R. What are the advantages and disadvantages of restructuring a health care system to be more focused on primary care services? London: Health Evidence Network. 2004.

Bach PB, Hoangmai H, Schrag D, Tate RC; Hargraves JL. Primary Care Physicians Who Treat Blacks and Whites. N Eng J Med. 2004;351: 575-584.

Baicker K, Chandra A. Medicare spending, the physician workforce, and beneficiaries' quality of care. Health Affairs (Millwood)(Suppl. Web Exclusives), 2004; W184–W197.

Bencho V, Schejbalova M. From Ignaz Semmelweis to the present: crucial problems of hospital hygiene. Indoor and Built Environment. 2006;15:3-8.

Bilcke J, Ogunjimi B, Marais C, et al. The health and economic burden of chickenpox and herpes zoster in Belgium. Epidemiol Infect. 2012;10:1-14.

BMA Board of Science and Education. Clinical hyperbaric medicine facilties in the UK London: BMA, 1993.

Boerma WGW and Fleming DM. The Role of General Practice in Primary Health Care. London: World Health Organization, 1998.

Boffetta P et al. Fruit and Vegetable Intake and Overall Cancer Risk in the European Prospective Investigation Into Cancer and Nutrition (EPIC). J Natl Cancer Inst. 2010; 102: 529-537.

Britton A, Brunner E, Kivimaki M, Shipley MJ. Limitations to functioning and independent living after the onset of coronary heart disease: what is the role of lifestyle factors and obesity? Eur J Public Health. 2011; doi: 10.1093/eurpub/ckr150.

Campbell JL, Medive J and Timmermans A. Primary care and general practice in Europe: West and South. In: Jones R, Britten N, Culpepper L et al (eds) Oxford Textbook of Primary Medical Care. Oxford: Oxford University Press, 2005, pp. 70–3.

Cegolon L, Miatto E, Bortolotto M, et al. *Body piercing and tattoo: awareness of health related risks among 4,277 Italian secondary school adolescents.* BMC Public Health. 2010a, 10:73

Cegolon L, Lange JH, Mastrangelo G. The Primary Care Practitioner and the diagnosis of occupational diseases. BMC Public Health. 2010b, 10:405

Center for Disease Prevention and Control (CDC, 2012). Alcohol & Public Health. Available at: www.cdc.gov/alcohol/ (accessed on 12 April 2012).

Centers for Disease Control. Pertussis outbreak among adults at an oil refinery--Illinois, August-October 2002. MMWR. 2003;10:1-4.

Chun Chen Y, Ching Wu J, Haschler I, Majeed A, Ji Chen T, Wetter T. Academic Impact of a Public Electronic Health Database: Bibliometric Analysis of Studies Using the General Practice Research Database. PLos One 2011; 6 (6): e21404.

David SP, Munafò MR. Smoking cessation in primary care. BMJ. 31 may 2008 | 336 1201. Cruz-Flores S, Rabinstein A, Biller J, Elkind MS, et al. Racial-ethnic disparities in stroke care: the American experience: a statement for healthcare professionals from the American Heart Association/American Stroke Association. Stroke. 2011 Jul;42(7):2091-116.

Day F, Sutton G. General practitioner notifications of gastroenteritis and food poisoning: cause for concern. J Public Health (Oxf). 2007;29:288-91.

Declaration of Alma-Ata. In International conference on primary health care, Alma-Ata, USSR. 1978.

De Macseneer J, Willems S. New Challenges Require New Types of Health Services Research. Abstract. Third bi-annual conference European Forum for Primary Care: The Future of Primary Health Care in Europe III, 2010.

Ebbert JO, Yang P, Vachon CM, Vierkant RA, Cerhan JR, Folsom AR, Sellers TA. Lung Cancer Risk Reduction After Smoking Cessation: Observations From a Prospective Cohort of Women. J Clin Oncol. 2003; 21:921-926.

Engstrom S, Foldevi M, Borgquist L. Is general practice effective? A systematic literature review. Scandinavian Journal of Primary Health Care. 2001; 19,131–144.

Ezzati M, Lopez AD, Rodgers A. Vander Hoorn, S., Murray, C. J., Selected major risk factors and global and regional burden of disease. Lancet. 2002. 360:1347-60.

Foxcroft DR , Ireland D, Lister-Sharp DJ, Lowe G, Breen R. Longer-term primary prevention for alcohol misuse in young people: a systematic review. Addiction. 2003; 98:397-411.

Franks P, Fiscella K. Primary care physicians and specialists as personal physicians. Health care expenditures and mortality experience. Journal of Family Practice. 1998; 47: 105–109.

Garrod ANI, Rajan Sithamparanadarajah R: Developing COSHH Essentials: Dermal Exposure, Personal Protective Equipment and First Aid. Ann Occup Hyg 2003. 47:577-588.

Gehle KS, Crawford JL, Hatcher MT. Integrating environmental health into medical education. Am J Prev Med. 2011;41(4 Suppl 3):S296-301.

Glasgow N. Systems for the management of respiratory disease in primary care - an international series: Australia. Prim Care Respir J. 2008;17:19-25.

Gollust S, Schroeder S, Warner K. Helping smokers quit: understanding the barriers to utilization of smoking cessation services. The Millbank Quarterly. 2008;86:601-27.

Gress S, Baan CA, Calnan M et al. Co-ordination and management of chronic conditions in Europe: the role of primary care. Position paper of the European Forum for Primary Care. Quality in Primary Care. 2009;17:75–86.

Groenewegen PP. Nursing as grease in the primary care innovation machinery. Quality in Primary Care. 2008;16:313–14.

Hajek P, Stead LF, West R, Jarvis M, Lancaster T. Relapse prevention interventions for smoking cessation (Review). The Cochrane Library. 2009; Issue 1. Available at: www.thecochranelibrary.com (accessed on 9 July 2010).

Hannay DR. Primary care and public health. BMJ. 1993; 307: 516-517.

Harris JR, Huang Y, Hannon PA, Williams B. Low-socioeconomic status workers: their health risks and how to reach them. J Occup Environ Med. 2011;53:132-8.

Health Council of the Netherlands. European primary care. The Hague. 2004.

Health and Safety Executive (HSE). COSHH Essentials--easy steps to control chemicals (HSG 193). Sudbury: HSE Books; 1999. ISBN 0 717.

Hajat S, O'Connor M, Kosatsky T. Health effects of hot weather: from awareness of risk factors to effective health protection. The Lancet. 2010; 375: 856–63.

Hobhom U. Toward general prophylactic cancer vaccination. Bioessays. 2009;31:1071-9.

Hogg W, Huston P, Martin C, Soto E. Enhancing public health response to respiratory epidemics: are family physicians ready and willing to help? Can Family Physician. 2006;52:1254-60.

Hu FB. Globalization of diabetes: the role of diet, lifestyle, and genes. Diabetes Care. 2011;34:1249-57.

Hughes JR, Peters EN, Naud S. Relapse to Smoking After 1 Year of Abstinence: A Meta-analysis. Addict Behav. 2008; 33: 1516–1520.

Hung HC, Joshipura KJ, Hu FB, et al. Fruit and Vegetable Intake and Risk of Major Chronic Disease. J Nat Cancer Inst. 2004; 96: 1577-84.

Keatinge WR. Death in heat waves. BMJ. 2003; 327: 512–13.

Katzmarzyk PT, Church TS, Blair SN. Cardiorespiratory fitness attenuates the effects of the metabolic syndrome on all-cause and cardiovascular disease mortality in men. Arch Intern Med. 2004;164:1092-7.

Kekki, P. Primary health care and the millennium development goals: Issues for discussion. Helsinki: University of Helsinki. 2006.

Khan K, McNabb SJ, Memish ZA, et al. Infectious disease surveillance and modelling across geographic frontiers and scientific specialties. Lancet Infect Dis. 2012:12:222-30.

Kruk ME, Porignon D, Rockers PC, Van Lerberghe W. The contribution of primary care to health and health systems in low- and middle-income countries: A critical review of major primary care initiatives. Social Science & Medicine 70 (2010) 904–911.

La Dou J. Current Occupational and Environmental Medicine . 4th edition. McGraw-Hill Publishers, New York, NY; 2008.

Lam DW, Le Roith D. The worldwide diabetes epidemic. Curr Opin Endocrinol Diabetes Obes. 2012;19:93-6.

Lange JH. SARS, emerging diseases, healthcare workers and respirators. J Hosp Infect. 2005;60:293.

Lange JH, Mastrangelo G, Cegolon L. Asbestos abatement workers versus asbestos workers: exposure and health-effects differ. Int J Occup Med Environm Health 2011; 24:418-9.

The Lancet (Editorial). Stemming the global tsunami of cardiovascular disease. The Lancet. 2011. 377 (February 12): 529-532.

Lau JT, Griffiths S, Choi KC, Lin C. Prevalence of preventive behaviors and associated factors during early phase of the H1N1 influenza epidemic. Am J Infect Control. 2010;38:374-80.

Levy TD, Graham AL, Mabry PL, Abrams DB, Orleans TB. Modeling the Impact of Smoking-Cessation Treatment Policies on Quit Rates. Am J Prev Med. 2010; 38(3S): S364-S372.

Liss GM, Buyantseva L, Luce CE, et al. Work-related asthma in health care in Ontario. Am J Ind Med. 2011;54:278-84.

Macinko J, Starfield B, Shi L. The contribution of primary care systems to health outcomes within Organization for Economic Cooperation and Development (OECD) countries, 1970–1998. Health Services Research. 2003; 38: 831–865.

Majeed A. Sources, uses, strengths and limitations of data collected in primary care in England. Health Statistics Quarterly 2004; 21: 5–14.

Medicine and Health Care Products Regulatory Agency. GPRD. Available at: http://www.gprd.com/home/

Morrell DC. Role of research in development of organisation and structure of general practice. BMJ. 1991;302:1313-6.

Mills M. Individualization and the life course: towards a theoretical model and empirical evidence. In: Howard C (ed) Contested Individualization: political sociologies of contemporary personhood. Basingstoke: Palgrave MacMillan, 2007: 61–79.

Mitchell JA, Bornstein DB, Sui X, et al. The impact of combined health factors on cardiovascular disease mortality. Am Heart J. 2010;160:102-8.

NHS (2010). What is a PCT? NHS Walsall. Available at: www.walsall.nhs.uk/about_us/whatisapct.asp (accessed on 7 February 2012).

New Zealand Health Information Service. Mortality and Demographic Data 2002 and 2003. Ministry of Health. 2006; available at: http://www.nzhis.govt.nz/moh.nsf/pagesns/528 (accessed on 15 Jan 2012).

Norval M, Lucas RM, Cullen AP, et al. The human health effects of ozone depletion and interactions with climate change. Photochem Photobiol Sci. 2011;10:199-225.

Orleans CT. Increasing the demand for and use of effective smoking-cessation treatments reaping the full health benefits of tobacco-control science and policy gains — in our lifetime. Am J Prev Med. 2007;33(6S):S340-8.

Orrow G, Kinmonth AL, Sanderson S et al., Effectiveness of physical activity promotion based in primary care: systematic review and meta-analysis of randomized controlled trials. BMJ. 344:e1389.

Piterman L, Koritsas S. Part I; General practitioner-specialist relationship. Intern Med 2005;35:430-4.

Preisig M, Waeber G, Mooser V, Vollenweider P. PsyCoLaus: mental disorders and cardiovascular diseases: spurious association? Rev Med Suisse. 2011; 7: 2127-9.

Reaven GM. Insulin resistance: the link between obesity and cardiovascular disease. Med Clin North Am. 2011 95:875-92.

Rosenblatt RA. Ecological change and the future of the human species: can physicians make a difference? Ann Fam Med. 2005;3:173-6.

Rosamond WD, Chambless LE, Heiss G, Mosley TH, Coresh J, Whitsel E, Wagenknecht L, Ni H, Folsom AR. Twenty-Two Year Trends in Incidence of Myocardial Infarction, CHD Mortality, and Case-Fatality in Four US Communities, 1987 to 2008. Circulation. 2012 Mar 15. [Epub ahead of print].

Sablan B. An update on primary care management for tuberculosis in children. Curr Opin Pediatr. 2009;21:801-4.

Schafer W. Groenewegen PP, Hansen J, Black N. Priorities for health services research in primary care. Quality in Primary Care. 2011;19:77–83.

Schneeweiss S, Avorn J. A review of uses of health care utilization databases for epidemiologic research on therapeutics. J Clinical Epid. 2005; 58:323–33.

Schulze MB, Hu FB. Primary prevention of diabetes: what can be done and how much can be prevented? Ann Rev Public Health. 2005:26:445-67.

Seidell JC, Flegal KM. Assessing obesity: classification and epidemiology. Br Med Bull. 1997;53:238-52.

Semenza JC, Suk JE, Estevez V, et al. Mapping Climate Change Vulnerabilities to Infectious Diseases in Europe. Environ Health Perspect. 2011;120:385-92.

Starfield B, Shi L, Macinko, J. Contribution of primary care to health systems and health. Milbank Q. 2005: 83:457–502.

Starfield B. Public Health and Primary Care: A Framework for Proposed Linkages. American Journal of Public Health. 1996; 86:1365-89.

Starfield, B. Primary care: Concept, evaluation, and policy. New York: Oxford niversity Press.1992.

Statistics Canada. Available at: www.statcan.gc.ca (accessed on 19 August 2010; updated on 3rd Feb 2009).

Statistics Netherlands. Cancer number one cause of death in 2008. Available at: www.cbs.nl/enGB/menu/themas/gezondheidwelzijn/publicaties/artikelen/arch ief/2009/2009-2687-wm.htm (Accessed on 19 August 2009; updated on 3 February 2009).

U.S. National Center for Health Statistics. Death by major causes, 1960-2005. National Vital Statistics Reports. 2006, vol.54 (19). Available at:
http://www.infoplease.com/ipa/A0005124.html (accessed on 12 July 2010).

UICC (2005). Cancer can be prevented too. Available at:
http://www.worldcancercampaign.org/index.php?option=com_content&task=vie w&id=273&Itemid=586 (accessed on 15 Jan 2012).

Uiters E, Deville W, Foets M, et al. Differences between immigrant and non-immigrant groups in the use of primary medical care; a systematic review. BMC Health Services Research. 2009;9:76.

UK Faculty of Public Health Medicine. UK levels of health. London: FPHM, 1992.

Van Weel C, Schers H, Timmermans A. Health care in the Netherlands. Am Board Fam Med 2012;25 (Suppl 1):S12-7.

Venkat A, Hunter R, Hegde GG, et al. Perceptions of Participating Emergency Nurses Regarding an ED Seasonal Influenza Vaccination Program. J Emerg Nurs. 2012;38:22-9.

Villalbi, JR, Guarga A, Pasarin MI, et al. An evaluation of the impact of primary care reform on health. Aten Primaria. 1999; 24:468 474.

Wagner KH, Brath H. A global view on the development of non communicable diseases. Prev Med. 2011 [Epub ahead of print].

Weevers HJ, van der Beek AJ, Anema JR, et al. Work-related disease in general practice: a systematic review. Fam Pract. 2005;22:197-204.

Welch WP, Miller ME, Welch HG, et al. Geographic variation in expenditures for physicians' services in the United States. New England Journal of Medicine, 1993; 328:621–627.

WHO (2012). Metrics: Disability-Adjusted Life Year (DALY). Health Statistics and Health Information Systems. Available at: www.who.int/healthinfo/global_burden_disease/metrics_day/en/ (accessed on 7 February 2012).

WHO (2011). Mortality, Cardiovascular diseases and diabetes, deaths per 100,000. Global Health Observatory Data Repository. Available at: www.who.int/ghodata/?vid=10011 (accessed on 7 February 2012).

WHO (2008). Integrating mental health into primary care: A global perspective. Geneva: WHO. whqlibdoc.who.int/publications/2008/9789241563680_eng.pdf (accessed on April 4, 2012).

WHO (2008a) The world health report. primary health care: now more than ever. Available at: http://books.google.it/books?hl=it&lr=&id=q-EGxRjrIo4C&oi=fnd&pg=PR8&dq =who+primary+care+more+than+ever&ots=YbrEXUILFp&sig=LpiHNS75aXP-oaTM6oOSKRVoitE#v=onepage&q=who%20primary%20care%20more%20than%2 0ever&f=false (accessed on 15 January 2012).

WHO (2008b). World Health Report 2008: Primary health care – Now more than ever. Geneva: WHO. www.who.int/whr/2008/en/index.html (accessed April 4, 2012)

WHO. Global burden of disease (2004 update). Available at: http://www.who.int/healthinfo/global_burden_disease/GBD_report_2004update _full.pdf (accessed on 15 Jan 2012).

WHO Europe 2004. Highlights on Heath in France. Available at: http://www.euro.who.int/__data/assets/pdf_file/0020/103853/E88547.pdf (accessed on 15 Jan 2012),

WHO Global Infobase: proportional mortlality. Available at: https://apps.who.int/infobase/Mortality.aspx (accessed on 15 Jan 2012).

WHO (2012a). Workplace Health Promotion. Available at: http://www.who.int/occupational_health/topics/workplace/en/ (accessed on 15 Jan 2012).

WHO (2000). World health report: health systems improving performance. Geneva, Switzerland. Available at: http://www.who.int/whr/2000/en/ (accessed on 15 Jan 2012).

Wiehe SE, Garrison MM, Christakis DA, Ebel BE, Rivara FP. A systematic review of school-based smoking prevention trials with long-term follow-up. J Adolesc Health. 2005;36:162–9.

Wilkinson RG. Income distribution and mortality: a 'natural' experiment. Sociol Health Illness. 1990;12:391-412.

Winchester CC, Macfarlane TV, Thomas M, Price D. Antibiotic prescribing and outcomes of lower respiratory tract infection in UK primary care. Chest. 2009;135:1163-72.

Windak A and Van Hasselt P.Primary care and general practice in Europe: Central and East. In: Jones R, Britten N, Culpepper L et al (eds) Oxford Textbook of Primary Medical Care. Oxford: Oxford University Press, 2005: 70–3.

Wong SY, Wong W, Jaakkimainen L, et al. Primary care physicians in Hong Kong and Canada--how did their practices differ during the SARS epidemic? Fam Pract. 2005;22:361-6.

2

At the Frontlines: Confronting Poverty in Primary Care Medicine

Namrata Kotwani, Ruqayyah Abdul-Karim and Marion Danis
Department of Bioethics, National Institutes of Health
USA

1. Introduction

1.1 Poverty and health

The effect of poverty on health status has been well-documented since the 1830s (Barnes, 1995; Engels, 1969; Poor Law Commissioners, 1842) and recent public health literature, especially since the 1970s, is replete with research which shows that the risk of developing disease appears to be related to socio- economic position (Hein et al., 1992; Hemingway et al., 2000; Marmot et al., 1978a; Marmot et al., 1978b; Rose & Marmot, 1981; Smith et al., 1997; Smith et al., 1998; WHO 2008). Moreover, a patient's uptake of preventative health recommendations and the success of a variety of chronic and acute therapeutic regimens are linked to socio-economic status. While socio-economic position affects health status continuously all along the socio-economic ladder, individuals living below the poverty line across the globe, have particularly dire health deficits. While these health deficits are largely the result of socio-economic factors that must be addressed through interventions that go beyond the bounds of the health care sector (CSDH, 2008), there are nonetheless a number of strategies that primary care providers can adopt to mitigate the effects of poverty on health.

1.2 Defining poverty

Definitions of poverty are varied and extend well beyond income to include inequities in the distribution of goods and services and the chance of leading a flourishing life. While consensus has not been reached on a standard definition of poverty, many global organizations have weighed in. The World Bank defines poverty as:

"[A] pronounced deprivation in well-being, and comprises many dimensions. It includes low incomes and the inability to acquire the basic goods and services necessary for survival with dignity. Poverty also encompasses low levels of health and education, poor access to clean water and sanitation, inadequate physical security, lack of voice, and insufficient capacity and opportunity to better one's life"(World Bank, 2000).

The United Nations developed a similar definition for poverty, which also touches on themes of living with dignity, a lack of capacity to meaningfully engage in society, and the inability to provide for basic social needs. Poverty is "sustained or chronic deprivation of the resources, capabilities, choices, security and power necessary for the enjoyment of an adequate standard of living" which creates conditions in which individuals are left vulnerable to crime and disease (UNESCO, 1998; United Nations Committee on Social, Economic and Cultural Rights, 2001). The international poverty line as set by the World Bank is defined as individuals living on $1.25 per day (World Bank, 2008), though the definition varies from country to country.

1.3 Prevalence of poverty

Poverty is a global phenomenon affecting low, middle, and high income countries. In the US, for example, where the government defines the poverty threshold as an income of $22,314 a year for a family of four and $11,139 for an individual, the Census Bureau's 2010 data indicated that 46.2 million people, comprising 15.1% of the population, were living in poverty (DeNavas-Walt et al., 2011). Table 1 shows country rankings and the percentage of the population in poverty in countries around the world (CIA World Factbook, 2011). Between 1990 and 2005, the number of people living below the international poverty line declined from 1.8 billion to 1.4 billion. The UN Millennium Development group has reported that overall poverty rates fell from 46 per cent in 1990 to 27 per cent in 2005 in developing regions, and progress in many developing countries is being sustained. Despite these advances, roughly 920 million people will still be living under the international poverty line by 2015 (UNDP, 2011). In a global climate of recession, this number would be likely to increase.

In many countries the prevalence of poverty is higher among ethnic and racial minorities and among immigrants than it is among those in the ethnic majority and native born population, although the pattern varies from country to country. In the United States African Americans and Latinos have much higher rates of poverty and tend to live in highly segregated housing as a result of a long history of discrimination that has been difficult to overcome (LaVeist 2005). In Canada by contrast, ethnic and minority groups are not as segregated into ghettos (Walks & Bourne, 2006). To the extent that poverty is associated with minority and immigrant populations, clinicians need to be sensitive to the deficits in health status and health care access of these populations.

1.4 Relationship of poverty to health

While this chapter focuses on the provision of primary care to the poor who are at the extreme low end of the socio-economic spectrum, a general understanding of the mechanisms underlying the social determinants of health is warranted to fully understand the needs of poor patients. The socio-economic determinants generally considered to be important include income, employment, education, housing and environment, nutrition, social support, and social inclusion (Lahelma et al., 2004). While personal behavior, such as smoking and alcohol, consumption, contribute to health, socio-economic factors are strongly associated with health even after adjusting for these personal behaviors (Lantz et al., 1998).

Several mechanisms have been postulated as mediating the influence of these socio-economic factors on health. Evidence of the biological pathways mediating the influence of socio-economic factors suggests that stress induced by social circumstances chronically stimulates the hypothalamic-pituitary-adrenal axis causing persistent adrenal hormones

Rank	Country	Pop. below poverty line (%)	Rank	Country	Pop. below poverty line (%)	Rank	Country	Pop. below poverty line (%)
1	Chad	80	36	Belize	43	71	Turkmenistan	30
2	Haiti	80	37	Dominican Republic	42.2	72	Virgin Islands	28.9
3	Liberia	80	38	Djibouti	42	73	Macedonia	28.7
4	Congo, Democratic Republic of	71	39	Cote d'Ivoire	42	74	Ghana	28.5
5	Sierra Leone	70.2	40	East Timor	42	75	Lebanon	28
6	Mozambique	70	41	Angola	40.5	76	Belarus	27.1
7	Nigeria	70	42	Bangladesh	40	77	Micronesia, Federated States of	26.7
8	Suriname	70	43	Sudan	40	78	Armenia	26.5
9	Gaza Strip	70	44	Mauritania	40	79	Moldova	26.3
10	Swaziland	69	45	Kyrgyzstan	40	80	Laos	26
11	Zimbabwe	68	46	Ethiopia	38.7	81	Brazil	26
12	Burundi	68	47	Venezuela	37.9	82	Uzbekistan	26
13	Honduras	65	48	El Salvador	37.8	83	Panama	25.6
14	Zambia	64	49	Benin	37.4	84	Fiji	25.5
15	Niger	63	50	Papua New Guinea	37	85	Iraq	25
16	Rwanda	60	51	Mongolia	36.1	86	India	25
17	Comoros	60	52	Mali	36.1	87	Romania	25
18	Guatemala	56.2	53	Tanzania	36	88	Nepal	24.7
19	Namibia	55.8	54	Afghanistan	36	89	Tonga	24
20	Senegal	54	55	Uganda	35	90	Pakistan	24
21	Sao Tome and Principe	54	56	Ukraine	35	91	Israel	23.6
22	Tajikistan	53	57	Peru	34.8	92	Bhutan	23.2
23	Malawi	53	58	Ecuador	33.1	93	Sri Lanka	23
24	Madagascar	50	59	Philippines	32.9	94	Algeria	23
25	Kenya	50	60	Burma	32.7	95	Anguilla	23
26	South Africa	50	61	Grenada	32	96	Guam	23
27	Eritrea	50	62	Togo	32	97	Bulgaria	21.8
28	Lesotho	49	63	Georgia	31	98	Slovakia	21
29	Nicaragua	48	64	Cambodia	31	99	Uruguay	20.9
30	Cameroon	48	65	Bolivia	30.3	100	Greece	20
31	Guinea	47	66	Botswana	30.3	101	Egypt	20
32	Burkina Faso	46.4	67	Argentina	30	102	Spain	19.8
33	West Bank	46	68	Cape Verde	30	103	Estonia	19.7
34	Colombia	45.5	69	Dominica	30	104	United Arab Emirates	19.5
35	Yemen	45.2	70	Kosovo	30	105	Bermuda	19

Rank	Country	Pop. below poverty line (%)	Rank	Country	Pop. below poverty line (%)	Rank	Country	Pop. below poverty line (%)
106	Paraguay	18.8	122	Korea, South	15	138	Canada	9.4
107	Bosnia and Herzegovina	18.6	123	Jordan	14.2	139	Bahamas, The	9.3
108	Mexico	18.2	124	United Kingdom	14	140	Greenland	9.2
109	Portugal	18	125	Hungary	13.9	141	Serbia	8.8
110	Iran	18	126	Indonesia	13.33	142	Kazakhstan	8.2
111	Turkey	17.11	127	Russia	13.1	143	Mauritius	8
112	Trinidad and Tobago	17	128	Albania	12.5	144	Montenegro	7
113	Poland	17	129	Slovenia	12.3	145	Switzerland	6.9
114	Croatia	17	130	Denmark	12.1	146	France	6.2
115	Jamaica	16.5	131	United States	12	147	Austria	6
116	Maldives	16	132	Syria	11.9	148	Ireland	5.5
117	Costa Rica	16	133	Chile	11.5	149	Lithuania	4
118	Japan	15.7	134	Azerbaijan	11	150	Tunisia	3.8
119	Germany	15.5	135	Vietnam	10.6	151	Malaysia	3.6
120	Belgium	15.2	136	Netherlands	10.5	152	China	2.8
121	Morocco	15	137	Thailand	9.6	153	Taiwan	1.16

Source: (CIA World Factbook, 2011)

Table 1. Country Rankings with Percentage of Population Living in Poverty

levels that predispose to obesity, diabetes, cardiovascular disease, and altered immune modulation (Brunner & Marmot, 2006). Another analytic strategy takes a life course approach building on evidence that a person's social circumstances at each point in time accumulate over a lifetime to contribute to an individual's health status so that, repeated periods of nutritional deficiency and social factors beginning in utero and running through childhood and adult life set up a sequence of poor development of the fetus, running through childhood and adult life leading to physiological damage and premature death in middle and early old age (Blane, 2006). There is also evidence that social support and social cohesion contribute to health and deficits in such support can affect physical and psychological morbidity as well as mortality (Stanfeld, 2006).

The poor are exposed to greater personal and environmental health risks, are less well nourished, have less information and are less able to access health care than those in higher socio-economic position; they thus have a higher risk of illness and disability. Conversely, illness can reduce household savings, lower learning ability, reduce productivity, and lead to a diminished quality of life, thereby perpetuating or even increasing poverty (WHO, 2008)

Those living in poverty have a lower life expectancy. One third of deaths - some 18 million people a year or 50,000 per day - are due to poverty-related causes. According to the World Health Organization, hunger and malnutrition are the single gravest threats to the world's public health; malnutrition is by far the biggest contributor to child mortality, being present in half of all cases of pediatric death (WHO, 2008). In the United States, the number of deaths attributed to socioeconomic health determinants, such as poverty, has been shown to be comparable to the number attributed to pathological and behavioral causes. In 2000, approximately 245,000 deaths were attributed to low education, 162,000 to low social support (comparable to the 155,000 lung cancer deaths that year), and 133,000 to individual-level poverty (Galea et al., 2011).

Living in a state of poverty can impede access to both primary and emergency care. People living in poverty have the greatest needs and face considerable challenges in obtaining medical treatment. According to the Canadian Community Health Survey, among Canadians with the lowest incomes, 40% suffer from chronic illnesses (Statistics Canada, 1997). People living in households with incomes under $20,000 are three times more likely to experience a decline in health status than those at higher income levels (Orpana HM, 2007). In one study, lower-income families were much likely to report delayed or foregone medical care because of issues related to the cost of care (Kullgren et al., 2010). This is further aggravated by a disconnect between physicians and their patients over the lived reality of poverty, which creates structural, attitudinal, and knowledge-based barriers to addressing poverty as a risk-factor to patient health (Bloch, 2011).

2. Addressing poverty in primary care

In this section of the chapter, we focus on evidence-based recommendations about adjustments in clinical practice that may significantly improve care for low-income individuals in the primary care setting (Table 2). While medical care alone cannot address the impact of low income, inadequate educational attainments, suboptimal living and work conditions, and material and other psychosocial deprivation on the health of patients, if physicians acknowledge the impact of these factors on their patients' health, they can utilize a range of therapeutic options to help their most disadvantaged patients.

When clinicians ignore the effects of poverty on health, they reduce their ability to improve the health status of a large fraction of the public, given how prevalent poverty is. Primary care clinicians can enhance clinical care and improve health outcomes for poor populations in ambulatory settings if they incorporate considerations about the socioeconomic status of patients within routine clinical practice. Marmot has proposed that the primary care clinician take a holistic approach to meeting the needs of poor patients that fully recognizes the full range of their needs (British Medical Association, 2011).

While the recommendations in this chapter are directed to primary care providers themselves, it is important to recognize that they will not have an opportunity to improve the health of poor patients unless patients have access to them and can respond to their interventions. Thus before considering how primary care providers can improve the care they offer, it is essential to consider larger structural issues. The Discussion paper for the 2011 World Conference on Social Determinants of Health considers the need to reorient health care services and public health programs to reduce inequities (WHO, 2011). As the document points out, to receive effective care, individuals need to know that they have a problem, seek care for this condition, gain access to care, receive appropriate advice, obtain the prescribed treatment, adhere to the treatment, and obtain effective relief from the treatment, with satisfactory resolution of their problem (WHO, 2011). To make these steps feasible health sector leadership must facilitate the funding, location, and timing of services and the competencies and attitudes of health workers. Health sector leaders must also work with communities to identify barriers and solutions, including ensuring that care extends beyond curative services to promotion and prevention activities. An essential ingredient to guaranteeing access to care is financing of equitable universally available health coverage (WHO, 2011).

Some of the most significant progress toward addressing poverty-related health deficits is likely to be accomplished through wide-scale governmental efforts. In the US, for example, where health disparities have been recognized to be a profound problem, the US Department of Health and Human Services (DHHS) outlined a series of interventions to address health care disparities building upon provisions in the Affordable Care Act of 2010 (US Department of Health and Human Services, 2011). In the European Union, DETERMINE is an EU Consortium for Action on the Socio-economic Determinants of Health (SDH) (2007 - 2010) aimed at increasing awareness and capacity among decision makers in all policy sectors to take health and health equity into consideration and to strengthen collaboration between health and other sectors. A summary of actions taken in various member states of the EU is available (Institute of Public Health in Ireland, 2010). The World Health Organization has made a number of recommendations for countries that seek to pursue similar efforts to address the socioeconomic determinants of health (Valentine et al., 2008).

2.1 Primary care interventions

Primary care physicians and other primary care providers (PCPs) are well positioned to educate low-income patients about the linkages between adverse life circumstances and poor health. PCPs often develop trusting relationships with their patients over the course of years, and enlarge their expertise in eliciting their patients' health goals and personal problems. Indeed, low-income patients may receive reliable health guidance only within the ambulatory care setting since their typical social milieu is characterized by poor health literacy, fragile support systems, and infrequent displays of ideal health behaviors. Here we enumerate a number of strategies (Table 2).

2.1.1 Screen and document poverty

It is not possible for clinicians to address the impact of poverty on health unless, they are aware of their patients' socio-economic status. While the literature does not yet provide a well established set of questions that clinicians should use to ascertain their patients' socio-economic status, some initial findings are worth attention. Measures of socio-economic status that have been shown to be good predictors of mortality are wealth and recent family income and they have been recommended for purposes of conducting research (Duncan et al., 2002). Primary care providers may find the results of a pilot study conducted in Canada more useful: the study found that a set of three questions were quite sensitive and specific for identifying poor patients in a family practice clinic: 'Have you (ever) had trouble making ends meet at the end of the month?'; "In the past year, was there any day when you or anyone in your family were hungry because you did not have enough money for food?; In the last month, have you slept outside, in a shelter, or in a place not meant for sleep? (Brcic et al., 2011)

Screen and document poverty	Incorporate questions about SES into screening questionnaires and into health records.
Appreciate impact of poverty on health status	Be familiar with the effects of socio-economic position on health status, health behavior, access to care, and response to interventions.
Correct organizational and logistical deficiencies	Use planned care visits for prevention activities. Distribute prevention activities among clinic staff as efficiently as possible. Ensure rapid availability of test results.
Formulate standard protocols for care delivery	Provide clinician prompts for screening tests, vaccines, and dietary counseling. Enable non-physician staff to deliver standard preventative care.
Provide extra outreach and assistance for vulnerable groups	Arrange point-of-service testing if feasible. Use intake questionnaires to elicit patient preferences and concerns. Extend nurse-managed chronic care supervision.
Support self-management	Send patient reminders through letters, voicemail, and email. Provide written treatment guides and dosage information. Address health literacy issues.
Evaluate intervention outcomes	Follow-up with patients using electronic disease management databases.
Address deficits in health status and health care access among ethnic minorities	Reduce discrimination Train staff to be sensitive to the needs of low-income and ethnic minority patients. Ensure availability of translators. Obtain feedback to measure quality of care.
Increase partnerships with agencies outside the healthcare system	Direct patients to government assistance programs, local educational resources, and advocacy organizations.
Educate patients about mitigating SEDH	Discuss the link between SES and disease. Acknowledge and address financial concerns.

Table 2. What can primary care physicians do to help their low-income patients?

2.1.2 Appreciate the affects of poverty on health

To most effectively help poor patients, it is useful for primary care clinicians to recognize the many ways that poverty predisposes patients to disease processes and shortens their life expectancy, and to also appreciate how the many deficits imposed by poverty make it more difficult for them to respond to therapeutic efforts.

Consider a young adult patient for example living in a poor community whose family lives in crowded housing in a neighborhood that has a high unemployment rate, high crime rate and few community resources. She did not finish high school because her family was unable to stay stably housed in one neighborhood and she found the stress of moving from one school to another so difficult that she could not keep up with schoolwork. She has been asked by her mother to help with the care of other children in the family. At 18 she was able to get a job at a fast food chain where she works part time. At age 24 she is overweight. She has felt overwhelmed with her extended family's situation and has little time to pay attention to health and has been embarrassed to deal with continued weight gain. At age 28, when she goes to the federally funded health clinic for treatment of a urinary tract infection, her primary care clinician finds that her fasting blood sugar is quite elevated. A repeat visit to the clinic when the infection is resolved reveals that the fasting blood sugar is high, the Hgb A1c level is 8.5, and the clinician tells her that she is diabetic. This young woman's primary care clinician will only be able to effectively help her once he or she appreciates that socioeconomic factors have clearly, over the course of her lifetime, had a cumulative effect on her health status and the likelihood that she will be able to pursue treatment for her obesity and diabetes, and preventive strategies to avoid cardiovascular disease.

2.1.3 Correct organizational and logistical deficiencies

The health care system is an important channel for reducing behavioral risk factors and increasing uptake of preventative strategies for low-income individuals. Thus, low-income patients can benefit enormously from the implementation of interventions that improve performance of indicated preventative activities in usual-practice settings. An evaluation of health care delivery systems in the US determined that hospital outpatient departments in particular offer high quality preventive services, due to benefit from institution-wide resources invested in systems to improve quality of care (Grossman et al., 2008). However, these benefits were limited by delays in health care and higher emergency room visits due access problems.

Impoverished patients consistently underutilize preventative health interventions such as adult immunizations and cancer screenings. For instance, the increasing rates of cancer deaths among low-income minority women can be partially attributed to lower screening rates and later detection of the disease. Black and Hispanic women, who are more vulnerable to poverty, have the lowest rates of cancer screening in the United States (Ramirez et al., 2000; Legler et al., 2002). Low-income patients tend to delay clinical contact until treatment is absolutely necessary because of the financial burden imposed by insurance co-payments, transportation costs, lost wages, and childcare arrangements. Thus, they are more likely to assume that the lack of obvious symptoms indicates absence of disease. A study of low-income minority women in community health centers showed that a large number would not undergo cancer screening since they did not experience any symptoms of ill health (Ogedegbe et al., 2005). The same study emphasized, however, that clinician recommendation was the most commonly cited encouragement for cancer screening among minority women. Data indicate that physicians miss several opportunities during office visits and acute care visits to help their patients avoid disease and serious complications through undertaking preventative care including vaccination, cancer screening, dietary counseling, and screening for chronic conditions such as diabetes and depression (Stone et al., 2002; Agency for Healthcare Research and Quality, 2006; Schmaling & Hernandez, 2005).

There are several ways of remedying these issues by correcting organizational and logistical deficiencies. Organizational changes in staffing and clinical procedures are most effective in improving rates of adult immunization and cancer screening (Stone, et al., 2002). Dramatic improvements in immunization and screening performance rates are possible through team-based quality improvement approaches and using planned care visits for prevention activities. In one example, a study sought to integrate an assessment of reproductive planning into the primary care encounter. This assessment was found to be important by 81% of the women surveyed (Dunlop et al., 2010) and it was found to be a useful tool in targeting individuals who were at high risk for unintended pregnancies. Another study in Appalachian Pennsylvania showed that colorectal cancer screening rates increased by 17% when physicians, nurses, and office staff were provided with information such as screening guidelines, county-specific cancer incidence and mortality data, and other educational tools (Curry et al., 2011). Such initiatives may redirect specific prevention activities to non-physician staff such as clerical or nursing staff that might identify patients needing prevention services and arrange physician visits, or enable nurses to utilize protocols to deliver preventive care themselves.

Having a usual source of care, especially a long relationship with a specific provider, is a strong predictor of adherence to prophylactic advice (Doescher et al., 2004). A survey of severely low-income Washington D.C. census tracts determined that if non-elderly women without a specific primary care physician were linked to a specific clinician at their primary care delivery site, adherence to Pap smear, clinical breast exam, and mammography by would increase by 30%, 15%, and 15% respectively (O'Malley et al., 2002). Reorganizing primary care services to boost continuous, longitudinal relationships with care providers may lead to significant strides in the success of health promotion interventions.

2.1.4 Formulate standard protocols for care delivery

Structured protocols for care delivery that allow bundling of appropriate intervention and health promotion strategies with comprehensive medical care may be particularly beneficial for low-income patients who are infrequent users of ambulatory care. Combining routine and preventive clinical care as a matter of standard practice ensures that patients will receive appropriate prophylactic care and education upon visiting a primary care clinic.

O'Malley et al. have demonstrated that low-income, inner-city women are more likely to adhere to cancer screening recommendations if a comprehensive array of services is available at the primary care delivery site (O'Malley et al., 2002). Similarly, physician prompts can also significantly increase the amount of educational and preventive care that patients receive. For instance, including health maintenance flow sheets on patient charts significantly increases vaccination rates among the elderly in diverse rural, inner-city, and suburban practices (Norwalk et al., 2004). Some patients are also more likely to engage in physical activity after physician-delivered tailored interventions (Dutton et al., 2007).

Increased uptake of disease-testing and screening among low socio-economic status (SES) patients is predicated on patient recall, convenience, and rapid availability of results (Warren et al., 2006). Outreach programs which generate quarterly reminders through letters, voicemail, and e-mail have been successful in persuading some individuals to schedule health screenings and self-management evaluations for chronic conditions. If feasible, providing point-of-service testing at primary care clinics would be a major convenience for low-income patients since it provides quick results and eliminates the need for repeat appointments. Point-of-service HIV testing in Baltimore City was found to have utility in groups at the highest risk of contracting the disease (Keller et al., 2011). In another study, however, only 81% of those testing positive returned for confirmatory results, compared to 91% of conventional test-takers (Guenter et al., 2008).

2.1.5 Provide extra outreach and assistance for vulnerable groups

The cumulative strain that accumulates from fighting challenging life circumstances often leaves poor patients unmotivated to deal with the cost and complexity of therapeutic regimens. While low-self efficacy may account for the inability of low-SES individuals to cope with medical problems, the systemic factors and provider attitudes which prevent them from self-managing diseases cannot not be ignored. Clinicians perceive their Medicaid patients, who typically belong to low SES, as less compliant than more affluent patients (Greene & Yedidia, 2005). Low-income patients also receive fewer referrals and fewer service options from their doctors.

Providers have fewer feelings of affiliation toward their low-income patients and are likely to underrate their likeability, competence, rationality, and self-control (Van Ryn & Burke et al., 2000). On average, physicians estimate that their lower SES patients are less likely to desire a physically active lifestyle or have a demanding career. Since disadvantaged patients may assign low priority to medical problems over other financial and social pressures, doctors might perceive such patients as non-compliant, unmotivated, and resistant to positive change (Reilly et al., 1998). Empirical evidence proves that facilitative provider behavior in the clinical setting is closely linked to improved physiological outcomes and self-management among low-income patients (Reilly et al., 1998). Physicians' negative attitudes toward low-income patients may hinder their ability to provide a clinical encounter that produces the best possible therapeutic outcomes. How can physicians provide the most facilitative clinical environment for their most disadvantaged patients?

Well-designed intake questionnaires can elicit patient expectations and preferences regarding illness and its management prior to physician contact. Such information allows the provider to allocate sufficient time for acute care, discussion of treatment plan and side-effects, patient education, and health promotion, which are key components of an optimal primary care visit. A key determinant of low-income patient satisfaction and health outcomes among low-income patients is the duration of the clinic visit (O'Malley et al., 2002B; Becker & Newsom, 2003). Further, Dugdale et al report that visit rates of above 3-4 per hour are associated with less data gathering, prevention, decreased patient satisfaction, increased patient turnover, and inappropriate prescribing (Dugdale et al., 1999). A Nigerian study in a resource-poor setting showed that increased time with clinicians combined with dietary education about caloric values of local food items reduced total morbidity for diabetes by half, in comparison to a control site where physician-patient interactions were not modified (Mshelia et al., 2007).

2.1.6 Support self-management

Self-management of chronic conditions may be especially difficult for low-income patients who may not be equipped to understand the complicated etiology of their disease and related coping strategies. Patient empowerment can be encouraged through the identification and acknowledgement of health literacy issues that limit patient understanding and compliance. Nearly 80 million US adults are thought to have limited health literacy, and rates are higher among the elderly, minorities, the uneducated, and the poor (Bennett et al., 2009; Kutner et al., 2006). Low rates of health literacy have been shown to be associated with poorer health outcomes, poorer use of health care services, and higher health costs overall (Berkman et al., 2011; Weiss et al, 1994). Interventions such as low-literacy health books provided to low-income parents of young children have been shown to reduce the number of emergency room and doctor visits, as well as the number of missed school and work days (Herman & Jackson, 2010).

Low levels of numeracy and literacy, common among low-income patients, might impede their ability to understand medication regimens and appropriate dosage. Although low-income patients are less likely to know the names of their medications, studies have shown that they are able to comply with medication schedules and dosages as well as more affluent patients (Kripalani et al., 2006). Research suggests that patients with low literacy may can learn and practice self-care behaviors with additional support and training (Pignone et al., 2006). Educational resources such as videotapes and other educational aids such as workbooks were highly valued by low-income patients suffering from anxiety disorders who found additional information about their condition to be "empowering"(Mukherjee et al., 2006).

Research shows that provider communication effectiveness and patient understanding are highly predictive of diabetes self-management (Heisler et al., 2002). This communication can be enhanced through the use of video-conferencing technology to overcome transportation-related obstacles in rural settings (Davis et al., 2010). Many low-income patients lack knowledge about their illness and its triggers and therefore, are unable to monitor and control their condition. For instance, poor inner-city asthmatic patients are less likely to understand exacerbation triggers, less likely to control their disease effectively, and more prone to emergency visits and hospitalization (Coyle et al., 2003). Patients would undoubtedly benefit from clear and concise written treatment guides which enumerate symptom triggers and management strategies in a simplified manner (Partridge, 2004).

2.1.7 Evaluate intervention outcomes

Team-based care coupled with aggressive case management could provide the consistent support and follow-up that patients from low-SES require. Data-driven care improvement for chronic disease management looks extremely promising in this regard. Developing electronic disease management databases enables physicians to follow-up with patients and track outcomes over time. A successful diabetes-management program maintained a computerized roster which included trends for major metabolic values, common co-morbidities, smoking status, and current medication for all patients (Kimura & Murkofsky, 2007). The roster was ranked so that high-risk patients were placed at the top and received more focused supervision such as reminders about regular follow-up visits, treatment regimen, and timely self-assessments. The greatest barrier to the widespread implementation of an electronic medical record system may be the cost burden placed on primary care practices in both high- and low-income countries (Holroyd-Leduc et al., 2011; Ludwick & Doucette, 2008).

Nurse-managed low-educated African American and Hispanic patients with systolic dysfunction reported fewer hospitalizations and better functioning (Sisk et al., 2006). These patients received guidance about diet, medication adherence, and self-management of symptoms through an initial visit and regularly scheduled follow-up telephone calls. Behavioral health specialists affiliated with a primary care provider served as care managers for economically disadvantaged patients suffering from panic disorder (Mukherjee et al., 2006). The specialists delivered cognitive behavioral therapy as an adjunct to physician prescribed pharmacotherapy, sought to increase adherence by calling patients who missed appointments, challenged negative beliefs among patients who were disinclined to pursue treatment, and relayed information about medication dosage and side-effect management.

2.1.8 Address deficits in health status and health care access among ethnic minorities

The 2011 report prepared by the US Department of Health and Human Services enumerated several ways that the primary care workforce can address health disparities among ethnic minority populations in the United States (US Department of Health and Human Services, 2011). The recommended strategies might be applicable to many nations where ethnic minorities experience health deficits relative to the remainder of the population. These recommendations include: making efforts to identify health disparities among racial and ethnic minorities; bridging language barriers for people whose primary language is not that of the native or dominant population and for whom the quality patient-provider interactions is likely to be inadequate by promoting the healthcare interpreting profession as an essential component of the healthcare workforce; enhance the cultural proficiency of the primary care workforce; incorporate community health workers into the primary care team to promote patient participation in health education, behavioral health education, prevention, and health insurance programs; increase the diversity of the healthcare and public health workforces since racial and ethnic minority practitioners are more likely to practice in medically underserved areas and provide health care to large numbers of racial and ethnic minorities (Komaromy 1996; Gonzales 1999; US Department of Health and Human Services, 2011).

Among primary care physicians practicing within the same large academic primary care system, patient panels with greater proportions of underinsured, minority, and non–English-speaking patients were associated with lower quality rankings for primary care physicians (Hong et al., 2010). At the same time, US physicians with a patient population that was over 50% Latino cited several hurdles to the delivery of high quality care to their patients, ranging from the patient's inability to pay to difficulties communicating because of language barriers (Vargas Bustamante & Chen, 2011). Low patient activation rates, which correlates with low skills, knowledge, confidence needed to properly manage one's own health, among Hispanic immigrants in the US was linked to low acculturation and lack of familiarity with the US healthcare system (Cunningham et al., 2011).

One way of directly addressing disparities due to ethnic differences is through the implementation of cultural competency training in medical education and practice. Such education enables medical students, staff and professionals to be sensitive to the needs of low-income patients. Interventions such as ensuring the availability of translators through a shared network of interpreter services is a cost-effective means of reducing barriers to communication between patients and their doctors without unduly burdening small practices and community health centers (Jacobs et al. 2011). A number of strategies have been shown to help reduce the tendency of medical trainees to unconsciously act in biased ways towards ethnic minority patients. In a review of these approaches, Woolf and Dacre report that discovering counter-stereotypical information about a patient, viewing a patient as having several social identities rather than one stereotyped identity, taking the patient's perspective, and seeing patient care as representing opportunities to put into practice one's goal of helping others can all help students avoid biased decision making and improve patient care (Woolf & Dacre, 2011).

2.1.9 Increasing partnerships with agencies outside the healthcare system

Several health care organizations have developed innovative programs that combine medical care with interventions that ameliorate disabling socioeconomic factors. For instance, the Orel Directly Observed Treatment Short course (DOTS) support program that operates in the Orel region of Russia recognizes that increased poverty and homelessness in the post-Soviet era are linked to the greater prevalence of tuberculosis (Ziglio et al., 2003). This program combines social support and medical treatment to promote adherence among impoverished TB patients and provides them with much-needed nutrition during recovery. In order to encourage patients to comply with DOTS therapy, food packages are given to patients each day they come to the clinic to take their medication. Nurses deliver food packages to elderly, infirm, or alcoholic TB sufferers who are unlikely to come to the clinic for their medication. Ensuring regular interaction with medical personnel and providing nutritional incentives has played a significant role in turning the Orel program into a model for successful tuberculosis control and management within resource-poor settings.

In a remarkable program located in Blackpool, England, general practitioners (GPs) observed that many of their patients displayed symptoms that stemmed from non-medical causes, often related to deteriorating local economic conditions (Ziglio et al., 2003). Patients were afflicted with sleeplessness, depression, and substance abuse, often linked to worries about indebtedness or other socioeconomic concerns. In order to assist patients to access non-medical resources, surgeries in the most deprived areas of Blackpool collaborated with the Citizens Advice Bureau (CAB), a national charity, to create a "one-stop shop" solution to medical, social, and psychological problems. Patient, who are generally poor, receive assistance in navigating the welfare system to claim a variety of benefits such as disability allowances, elder care supplements, and unemployment benefits and may also be provided debt counseling upon request. Staff members can be consulted at several GP surgeries and many patients are referred to them by medical personnel. This seamless integration of medical and social services allows the poor, elderly, and disabled patients to attain financial and mental security.

Similarly, "Just for Us" is another joint program run by an academic medical center and community organizations which provides financially sustainable, in-home, integrated care to frail low-income seniors and disabled adults living in subsidized housing (Yaggy et al., 2006). The stakeholders include a community health center, county social and mental health agencies, and a city housing authority, which coordinate services to promote the health and independence of these seniors. A multidisciplinary team provides in-home primary care and chronic disease management based on a fee-for-service model. Besides evidence-based medical care, the seniors receive assistance in obtaining Medicaid privileges, food stamps, and Meals on Wheels. Social workers provide intensive case management and services such as protective services (if abuse is discovered), post-hospitalization follow-up, assistance in obtaining durable medical equipment, mental health care and public transportation benefits. Costs for emergency department use and inpatient care, which are reliable indicators of the health status of elderly citizens, have dropped substantially.

Intensive case management for substance-dependent women receiving Temporary Assistance for Needy Families (TANF) has been shown to yield higher levels of substance abuse treatment initiation, engagement, retention, and higher likelihood of abstinence at 15-month follow- up (Morgenstern et al., 2006). Case managers addressed barriers to entry which included childcare, transportation, and housing problems. Additionally, they provided motivational counseling coupled with outreach methods such as home visits and contacting family members. Clients received incentives such as vouchers for purchasing children's toys and cosmetics for attending treatment.

A special unit for tuberculosis treatment in Hungary which targets homeless and alcoholic TB patients has dramatically curbed recidivism rates for disease and substance abuse by introducing a comprehensive program of recovery (Ziglio et al., 2003). Patients undergo therapy for alcoholism if necessary, and the primary problem of homelessness is addressed through an innovative re-housing program. Recovered patients are placed into housing established or financed by a foundation where they can stay for a period of 2-3 years. The recovered individuals find employment, contribute to common housing expenses, and save money to become financially solvent and slowly reintegrate into mainstream society.

The BfreeNYC screening program for Hepatitis B in low-income communities has been found to have a significant impact on the reduction of health disparities in communities of recent immigrants (Pollack et al., 2011). Stakeholders included members from the fields of community health, local government, academic institutions, public hospitals, and private physician practices. The program provided free community-based screenings, vaccinations, and care of Hepatitis B, and showed positive outcomes in program effectiveness and the reduction of morbidity and mortality.

2.1.10 Educate patients about mitigating SEDH

As noted earlier, it is possible for physicians to use brief intake questionnaires to quickly establish the patient's socio-economic status. By asking questions related to education and training, financial situation, employment, risky behaviors and addictions, a physician can learn about and, in turn, educate patients about specific socio-economic factors that impede the patient's well-being or hinder treatment adherence. Physician-directed conversations may help patients understand that their medical problems often have a social context.

Depending on their circumstances, patients could be referred to social welfare programs or local charitable organizations such as Women, Infants, and Children (WIC) supplemental nutritional services, alcohol and drug abuse treatment programs, domestic violence shelters, legal aid, community colleges, clergy, career counselors, employment agencies, homeless shelters, language training sites, community libraries, and other advocacy organizations for the underserved. Often physician endorsement of a particular intervention may eliminate the patient's initial inhibition or resistance to seeking proper assistance.

Returning to the newly diagnosed diabetic young woman introduced earlier, the various strategies can be usefully applied to her care along with the usually recommended approach strategies outlined here. According to standard recommendations, her primary care provider focuses on trying to manage her hyperglycemia as recommended by guidelines and explains the need for a diet, exercise and weight loss (Nathan et al., 2006; Nathan et al., 2009). She also aims to provide the recommended health maintenance for her patient (American Diabetes Association, 2011). She focuses on multi-factorial risk reduction to reduce the risk of coronary artery disease, including reducing dietary fat; Light to moderate exercise; Smoking cessation; Tight glycemic control (target A1C <6.5 percent with intensive therapy); Tight blood pressure control (target <140/85 mmHg for most of the study and <130/80 mmHg for the last two years); Angiotensin converting enzyme (ACE) inhibitor therapy regardless of blood pressure; Lipid-lowering therapy (target total cholesterol <190 mg/dL [4.9 mmol/L] for most of the study and <175 mg/dL [4.5 mmol/L] for the last two years; target fasting serum triglyceride <150 (Gaede et al., 2003).

These standards of care will not be effective, however, unless her primary care provider makes an effort to discover that the patient is poor, collects information about her social circumstances and understands her lived reality of poverty, and develops a care plan that takes this reality into account (Bloch, et al. 2011). Strategies recommended above including making available assistance with furthering her education, job training and employment services will be important aspects of holistic care to improve her situation (British Medical Association, 2011). Studies demonstrate a number of approaches that are specifically aimed at improving the successful management of poor diabetic patients including the use of physician-community health worker partnering to support diabetic self management (Otero-Saboquai et al, 2010); certified medical-assistance coaches with specific diabetes training (Ruggiero et al, 2010); literacy sensitive , culturally tailored, group-based self management interventions involving sessions to teach knowledge, attitudes and self-management behaviors (Rosal et al, 2011); and a telephone delivered physical activity and dietary intervention (Goode et al, 2011).

3. Barriers to improving primary care for low-income populations

Several obstacles must be overcome to facilitate primary care providers' efforts to ensure the best possible care to low-income patients. Bureaucratic obligations coupled with low reimbursement rates often force them to increase patient volume and abbreviate patient appointments (Larson et al., 2003). Consequently, clinicians primarily focus on acute problems and spend less time on patient education, disease prevention, and general health counseling. Since low-income patients derive the greatest marginal benefit from health education, personalization of treatment regimens, and motivational counseling, they stand to lose the most when face time with physicians is reduced. Current performance measure indicators have not recognized care coordination in the treatment of chronic conditions and time spent on health promotion activities (Larson et al., 2003).

Moreover, performance measures usually assess quality of care for specific diseases but cannot satisfactorily evaluate care that mitigates multiple, concurrent illnesses prevalent among low SES adults. Attaining quality goals among poorer patients is substantially more demanding than improving health outcomes for well-educated, materially privileged patients. Thus, aligning financial incentives with improved outcomes without provisions for measuring baseline health indicators may press doctors to avoid treating poor patient (Committee on quality Health Care in America, 2001). Since improvements in patient outcomes and quality goals can be attributed to the efforts of the entire care team, performance payments could be used to improve systems rather than reward individual physicians.

Lack of research also inhibits the ability to provide optimal care to disadvantaged patients. Although poverty and psychosocial deprivation has been linked conclusively to poorer health, intervention studies that determine the effect of combining conventional medical therapy with socioeconomic interventions have not been designed and evaluated to the same extent. Partnerships between academic medical center and community organizations may be ideal vehicles for the delivery and assessment of socioeconomic interventions. For instance, Stone et al point out that there is insufficient evidence to link increased uptake of preventative services among adults and financial incentives such as reduced co-payments and monetary compensation for adherence (Stone et al., 2002).

Clinical practice guidelines which incorporate socioeconomic evidence are uncommon (Aldrich et al., 2003). Systems change will likely be an effective way of streamlining care for low-SES patients. Rust and Cooper posit that organizational change in clinical setting resets the default setting from "don't do anything unless the doctor orders it" to "do automatically the evidence-based things the doctor would want to have done" (Rust & Cooper, 2007). Newer models of clinical organization could direct care through a multidisciplinary team including nurses (through protocols) and front-desk staff (providing age and gender appropriate health promotion materials, in addition to using time spent by patients in the waiting room (intake questionnaires, self-scoring depression or obesity scales, or disease specific kiosks). However, literature that evaluates the effectiveness of systems innovation in improving care for low-SES patients remains quite scanty.

4. Conclusions

While we have mentioned many strategies that primary care providers can employ to mitigate the impact of poverty on health, we acknowledge several limitations. A clinician working with an adult patient cannot undo the cumulative effects of poor nutrition, education, and housing experienced since childhood. Socioeconomic interventions thus are most likely to show profound improvements in overall well-being if they are introduced during childhood. Moreover, the success of many interventions enumerated above is contingent on organizational strategies and programs that individual clinicians can hardly muster alone. Most, although not all of the evidence-based interventions we have mentioned here, address the effects of poverty in developed countries such as the United States. The level of deprivation in the developing world is such that other infrastructural modifications such as the provision of clean water, clean air, and sewage disposal may be more productive as health improvement strategies.

Clearly, development of evidence-based strategies and design of delivery systems consistent with such evidence is needed to ensure that the most vulnerable and impoverished members of society benefit from primary care. In 2006, the National Healthcare Disparities Report recorded that poor people received worse quality of care than their affluent compatriots in 71 percent of care quality measures (Agency for Healthcare Research and Quality, 2006). Evidence indicates that primary health care, particularly when delivered effectively in combination with interventions that tackle socio-economic influences on health can improve the health of poor populations. Primary care clinicians should make every effort to put this evidence into practice.

5. Acknowledgment

The preparation and publication of this chapter was funded by the Department of Bioethics at the Clinical Center of the National Institutes of Health. The views expressed here are those of the authors and not necessarily a reflection of the policies of the National Institutes of Health or the US Department of Health and Human Services.

6. References

Agency for Healthcare Research and Quality. National Healthcare Quality Report, 2006. (2006) *Agency for Healthcare Research and Quality*, Rockville, MD. 2006. Available at from <http://www.ahrq.gov/qual/nhqr06/nhqr06.htm>.

Aldrich, R.; Kemp, L. & Williams, J.S. et al. (2003). Using socioeconomic evidence in clinical practice guidelines. *British Medical Journal*. Vol. 327, No. 7426, pp. 1283-1285.

American Diabetes Association. Standards of medical care in diabetes--2011. *Diabetes Care*. Vol. 34, pp. Suppl 1:S11.

Barnes, DS. (1995). *The Making of a Social Disease*. Berkeley, CA: University of California Press 1995.

Becker, G. & Newsom, E. (2003). Socioeconomic status and dissatisfaction with health care among chronically ill African Americans. *Am J Public Health*. Vol. 93, No. 5, pp. 742-748.

Bennett, I.M.; Chen, J.; Soroui, J.S. & White, S. (2009). The Contribution of Health Literacy to Disparities in Self-Rated Health Status and preventive Health Behaviors in Older Adults. *Annals of Family Medicine*. Vol. 7, No. 3, pp. 204-211.

Berkman, N.D.; Sheridan, S.L.; Donahue, K.E.; Halpern, D.J. & Crotty, K. (2011). Low Health Literacy and Health Outcomes: An Updated Systematic Review. *Annals of Internal Medicine*. Vol. 155, No. 2, pp. 97-107.

Bisgaier, J. & Rhodes, K.V. (2011). Access to specialty care for children with public versus private insurance. *N Engl J Med, Vol.* 364, pp. 2324-33.

Blane, D. (2006) The Life Course, the Social Gradient, and Health. In Marmot & Wilkinson (Eds.), *Social Determinants of Health,. Second Edition*. Oxford University Press, Oxford, UK.: Oxford University Press. 2006.

Bloch, G.; Rozmovits, L. & Giambrone, B. (2011). Barriers to primary care responsiveness to poverty as a risk factor for health. *BMC Family Practice.* Vol. 12, No. 62, pp. 1-6.

Brcic, V.; Eberdt, C. & Kaczorowski, J. (2011). Development of a tool to indentify poverty in a family practice setting: A pilot study. *International Journal of Family Medicine.* Vol. 2011, pp. 1-7.

British Medical Association. (2011). Social Determinants of Health: What Doctors Can Do. *British Medical Association.* 09-11-2011, Available from <http://www.bma.org.uk/images/socialdeterminantshealth_tcm41-209805.pdf>

Brunner, E. & and Marmot, M. (2006). Social Organization, stress, and health. In Marmot M & Wilkinson RG (Eds.), Social Determinants of Health, Second Edition. *Oxford University Press,* Oxford, UK.

CIA World Factbook. (2011). Field Listing: Population Below Poverty Line. *Central Intelligence Agency,* 09-11-2011, Available from, <https://www.cia.gov/library/publications/the-world-factbook/fields/2046.html >, ISSN 1553-8133.

Commission on Social Determinants of Health. (2008). Closing the gap in a generation: health equity through action on the social determinants of health. Final Report of the Commission on Social Determinants of Health. *World Health Organization,* Geneva. Available from <http://whqlibdoc.who.int/publications/2008/9789241563703_eng.pdf>

Committee on Quality Health Care in America. (2001). Crossing the Quality Chasm: a new health system for the 21st century. *Institute of Medicine,* Washington D.C. : Institute of Medicine, 2001.

Cooper-Patrick, L.; Gallo, J.J.; Gonzales, J.J.; Vu, H.T.; Powe, N.R.; Nelson, C. & Ford, D.E. (1999) Race, gender and partnership in the patient-physician relationship. *JAMA,* Vol. 282. No. 6, pp. 583-9.

Coyle, Y.M.; Aragaki, C.C.; Hynan, L.S.; Gruchalla, R.S. & Khan, D.A. (2003). Effectiveness of Acute Asthma Care Among Inner-city Adults. *Arch Intern Med.,* Vol. 163, No. 13, pp. 1591-1596.

Cunningham, P.J.; Hibbard, J. & Gibbons, C.B. (2011) Raising Low "Patient Activation" Rates Among Hispanic Immigrants May Equal Expanded Coverage In Reducing Access Disparities. *Health Affairs.* Vol. 30, No. 10, pp. 1888-1894.

Curry, W.J.; Lengerich, E.J.; Kluhsman, B.C.; Graybill, M.A.; Liao, J.Z.; Schaefer, E.W.; Spleen, A.M. & Dignan, M.B. (2011). Academic detailing to increase colorectal cancer screening by primary care practices in Appalachian Pennsylvania. *BMC Health Serv Res.* Vol. 11, No. 1, pp. 112.

Davis, R.M.; Hitch, A.D.; Salaam, M.M.; Herman, W.H.; Zimmer-Galler, I.E. & Mayer-Davis, E.J. (2010). TeleHealth Improves Diabetes Self-Management in an Underserved Community. *Diabetes Care.* Vol. 33, No. 8, pp. 1712-1717.

DeNavas-Walt, C.; Proctor, B.D. & Lee, C.H. (2011). Income, Poverty, and Health Insurance Coverage in the United States: 2010. *US Census Bureau.* pp. 60-231. Available from < http://www.census.gov/prod/2011pubs/p60-239.pdf>

Doescher M.P.; Saver B.G.; Fiscella, K. & Franks P. (2004) Preventive care: Does Continuity Count? *J Gen Intern Med.* Vol. 19, No. 6, pp. 632-637.

Dugdale, D.C.; Epstein, R. & Pantilat, S.Z. (1999). Time and the patient-physician relationship. *J Gen Intern Med*. Vol. 14, Suppl 1:, pp. S34-40.

Duncan GJ, Daley MC, McDonough P, Williams DP. (2002) Optimal indicators of socioeconomic status for health research. *American Journal of Public Health*. 92:1151-1157.

Dunlop, A.L.; Logue, K.M.; Miranda, M.C. & Narayan, D.A. (2010). Integrating reproductive planning with primary health care: an exploration among low-income, minority women and men. *Sex Reprod Healthc*. Vol. 1, No, 2, pp. 37-43.

Dutton, G.R.; Davis Martin, P.; Welsch, Michael A. & Brantley, P.J. (2007). Promoting Physical Activity for Low-income Minority Women in Primary Care. *Am J Health Behav*. Vol. 31, No. 6, pp. 622-631.

Engels, F. (1969) *Condition of the Working Class in England*. Panther, London, England: Panther 1969.

Gaede, P.; Vedel, P.; Larsen, N. et al. (2003). Multifactorial intervention and cardiovascular disease in patients with type 2 diabetes. *N Engl J Med*. Vol 348, pp. 383.

Galea, S.; Tracy, M.; Hoggart, K.; Dimaggio, C.; & Karpati, A. (2011). Estimated Deaths Attributable to Social Factors in the United States. *Am J of Pub Hlth*. Vol. 101, pp. 1456-1465.

Goode, A.D.; Winkler, E.A.; Lawler, S.P.; Reeves, M.M.; Owen, N. & Eakin, E.G. (2011) A telephone delivered physical activity and dietary intervention for type 2 diabetes and hypertension: does intervention dose influence outcomes?. *American Journal of Health Promotion*, Vol. 25, No. 4, pp. 257-263.

Great Britain. Poor Law Commissioner. (1842). Report to Her Majesty's Principal Secretary of State for the Home Department from the Poor-Law Commissioners on an Inquiry into the Sanitary Condition of the Labouring Population of Great Britain. *London: W. Clowes & Sons*, Available at from:
<http://www.victorianweb.org/history/chadwick2.html>.

Greene, J. & Yedidia, M.J. (2005). Provider behaviors contributing to patient self-management of chronic illness among underserved populations. *J Health Care Poor Underserved*. Vol. 16, No. 4, pp. 808-824.

Grossman, E.; Legedza, A.T.R. & Wee, C.C. (2008). Primary Care for Low-Income Populations: Comparing Health Care Delivery Systems. *J Hlth Care for the Poor and Underserved*. Vol. 19, pp. 743-757.

Hein, HO.; Suadicani, P. & Gyntelberg, F. (1992). Ischaemic heart disease incidence by social class and form of smoking: the Copenhagen Male Study--17 years' follow-up. *J Intern Med*. Vol. 231, No. 5, pp. 477.

Heisler, M.; Bouknight, R.R.; Hayward, R.A.; Smith, D.M., & Kerr, E.A. (2002). The relative importance of physician communication, participatory decision making, and patient understanding in diabetes self-management. *J Gen Intern Med.*, Vol. 17, No. 4, pp. 243-252.

Hemingway, H.; Shipley, M.; Macfarlane, P. & Marmot, M. (2000). Impact of socioeconomic status on coronary mortality in people with symptoms, electrocardiographic abnormalities, both or neither: the original Whitehall study 25 year follow up. *J Epidemiol Community Health*. Vol. 54, No. 7, pp. 510.

Herman, A. & Jackson, P. (2010). Empowering low-income parents with skills to reduce excess pediatric emergency room and clinic visits through a tailored low literacy training intervention. *J Health Commun.* Vol. 15, No. 8, pp. 895-910.

Hofer, A.N.; Abraham, J.M. & Moscovice, I. (2011). Expansion of coverage under the Patient Protection and Affordable Care Act and primary care utilization. *Milbank Q.* Vol. 89, No. 1, pp. 69-89.

Holyroyd-Leduc, J.M.; Lorenzetti, D.; Straus, S.E.; Sykes, L. & Quan, H. (2011) The impact of the electronic medical record on structure, process, and outcomes within primary care: a systematic review of the evidence. *J Am Med Inform Assoc.* Vol. 18, pp. 732-737.

Hong, C.S.; Atlas, S.J.; Chang, Y.; Subramanian, S.V.; Ashburner, J.M.; Barry, M.J. & Grant, R.W. (2010). Relationship Between Patient Panel Characteristics and Primary Care Physician Clinical Performance Rankings. *JAMA*, Vol. 304, No. 10, pp. 1107-1113.

Institute of Public Health in Ireland. (2010). Policies and actions addressing the socio economic determinants of health inequalities: Examples of activities in Europe. *Institute of Public Health in Ireland.* 09-11-2011, Available at: http://www.politiquessociales.net/IMG/pdf/DETERMINE.pdf

Kimura, J. &, Murkofsky, R.. (2007). Diabetes Dashboards - Bringing Population Management to Primary Care. SGIM Forum. 2007; Vol 30, No. (2).

Koh, H.K.; Graham, G. & Glied, S.A. (2011). Reducing Racial and Ethnic Disparities: The Action Plan from the Department of Health and Human Services. *Health Affairs.* Vol. 30, No. 10, pp. 1822-1829.

Lantz, P.M.; House, J.S.; Lepkowski, J.M.; Williams, D.R.; Mero, R.P.& Jieming Chen, J. (1998). Socioeconomic Factors, Health Behaviors, and Mortality: Results from a Nationally Representative Prospective Study of US Adults. *JAMA.* Vol. 279, No. 21, pp. 1703-1708.

Larson, E.,; Kirk, L., & Levinson, W,. et al. (2003). The Future of General Internal Medicine. *Society of General Internal Medicine,* Washington, D.C. : Society of General Internal Medicine, 2003. Available from <http:///www.sgim.org/futureofGIM.pdf>.

LaVeist TA. (2005) Socioeconomic status and Racial/Ethnic Differences in Health in *Minority Populations and Health* Josey Bass San Fransisco. pp. 157-179.

Legler, J.; Meissner, H.I.; Coyne, C.; Breen, N.; Chollette, V. & Rimer, B.K. (2002). The effectiveness of interventions to promote mammography among women with historically lower rates of screening. *Cancer Epidemiol Biomarkers Prev.* Vol. 11, No. 1, pp. 59-71.

Ludwick, D.A. & Doucette, J. (2009) Adopting electronic medical records in primary care: Lessons learned from health information systems implementation experiences in seven countries. *International Journal of Medical Informatics.* Vol. 78, pp. 22-31.

Marmot, M.G.; Adelstein, A.M.; Robinson, N. & Rose, G.A. (1978). Changing social-class distribution of heart disease. *Br Med J.* Vol. 2, No. 6145, pp. 1109.

Marmot, M.G.; Rose, G.; Shipley, M. & Hamilton, P.J. (1978). Employment grade and coronary heart disease in British civil servants. *J Epidemiology Community Health.* Vol. 32, No. 4, pp. 244.

Morgenstern, J.; Blanchard, K.A.; McCrady, B.S.; McVeigh, K.H.; Morgan, T.J. & Pandina, R.J. (2006). Effectiveness of intensive case management for substance-dependent women receiving temporary assistance for needy families. *Am J Public Health.* Vol. 96, No. 11, pp. 2016-2023.

Mshelia, D.S.; Akinosun, O.M. & Abbiyesuku, F.M. (2007). Effect of increased patient-physician contact time and health education in achieving diabetes mellitus management objectives in a resource-poor environment. *Singapore Med J.* Vol. 48, No. 1, pp. 74-79.

Mukherjee, S.; Sullivan, G. &, Perry, D., et al. (2006). Adherence to treatment among economically disadvantaged patients with panic disorder. *Psychiatr Serv.* Vol. 57, No. 12, pp. 1745-1750.

Nathan, D.M.; Buse, J.B.; Davidson, M.B. et al. (2006). Management of hyperglycemia in type 2 diabetes: A consensus algorithm for the initiation and adjustment of therapy: a consensus statement from the American Diabetes Association and the European Association for the Study of Diabetes. *Diabetes Care.* Vol. 29, pp. 1963.

Nathan, D.M.; Buse, J.B.; Davidson, M.B. et al. (2009). Medical management of hyperglycemia in type 2 diabetes: a consensus algorithm for the initiation and adjustment of therapy: a consensus statement of the American Diabetes Association and the European Association for the Study of Diabetes. *Diabetes Care.* Vol. 32, pp. 193.

Nowalk, M.P.; Zimmerman R.K. & Feghali, J. (2004). Missed opportunities for adult immunization in diverse primary care office settings. *Vaccine.* Vol. 22, No. 25-26, pp. 3457-3463.

Ogedegbe, G.; Cassells, A.N. & Robinson, C.M., et al. (2005). Perceptions of barriers and facilitators of cancer early detection among low-income minority women in community health centers. *J Natl Med Assoc.* Vol. 97, No. 2, pp. 162-170.

O'Malley A.S.; Forrest C.B. & Mandelblatt, J. (2002) Adherence of low-income women to cancer screening recommendations. *J Gen Intern Med.* Vol. 17, No. 2, pp. 144-154.

O'Malley, A.S. & Forrest, C.B. (2002). The mismatch between urban women's preferences for and experiences with primary care. *Womens Health Issues.* Vol. 12, No. 4, pp. 191-203.

Orpana, H.M.; Lemyre, L. & Kelly, S. (2007). Do stressors explain the association between income and declines in self-rated health? A longitudinal analysis of the National Population Health Survey. *Int J Behav Med,* Vol. 14, pp. 40-47.

Otero-Saboquai, R.; Arretz, D.; Siebold, S.; Lee, R.; Ketchel, A.; Li, J. & Newman, J. (2010). Physician-community health worker partnering to support diabetes self-management in primary care. *Quality Primary Care.* Vol. 18, pp. 363-372.

Partridge, M.R. (2004).Written asthma action plans. *Thorax.* 2004;Vol. 59(, No. 2):, pp. 87-88.

Pignone, M.P. &P, DeWalt, D.A. (2006). Literacy and health outcomes: is adherence the missing link? *J Gen Intern Med.*; Vol. 21, No. 8, (August 2006), pp. 896-897.

Pollack, H; Wang, S.; Wyatt, L.; Peng, C.; Wan, K.; Trinh-Shevrin, C.; Chun, K.; Tsang, T. & Kwon, S. (2011). A comprehensive screening and treatment model for reducing disparities in Hepatitis B. *Health Affairs.* Vol. 30, No. 10, pp. 1974-1983.

Ramirez, A.G.; Suarez, L.; Laufman, L.; Barroso, C. & Chalela, P. (2000). Hispanic women's breast and cervical cancer knowledge, attitudes, and screening behaviors. *Am J Health Promot.* Vol. 14, No. (5), pp. 292-300.

Reilly, B.M.; Schiff, G. &, Conway, T. (1998). Primary care for the medically underserved: challenges and opportunities. *Dis Mon.* Vol. 44, No. 7, (Jul 1998), pp. 320-346.

Rosal, M.C.; Ockene, I.S.; Restrepo, A.; White, M.J.; Borg, A.; Olendzki, B.; Scavron, J., Candib, L.; Welch, G. & Reed, G. (2011). Randomized trial of literacy-sensitive, culturally tailored diabetes self-management intervention for low-income latinos: latinos en control. *Diabetes Care,* Vol. 34, No 4, pp. 838-844.

Rose, G. & , Marmot, MG. (1981) Social class and coronary heart disease. *Br Heart J.* Vol. 1981;45, No. (1,):pp.13-19.

Ruggiero,L.; Moadsiri, A.; Butler, P.; Oros, S.M.; Berbaum, M.L.; Whitman, S. & Cintron, D. (2010). Supporting diabetes self-care in underserved populations: a randomized pilot study using medical assistant coaches. *Diabetes Education,* Vol. 36, No. 1, pp. 127-131.

Rust, G. & Cooper, L.A. (2007). How can practice-based research contribute to the elimination of health disparities? *J Am Board Fam Med.* 2007 Mar-Apr;Vol. 20, No, (2):, pp. 105-114.

Schmaling, K.B. & Hernandez, D.V. (2005). Detection of depression among low-income Mexican Americans in primary care. *J Health Care Poor Underserved.* 2005 Vol. Nov;16, No, (4):, pp. 780-790.

Sisk, J.E.; Hebert, P.L.; Horowitz, C.R.; McLaughlin, M.A.; Wang, J.J. & Chassin, M.R. (2006). Effects of nurse management on the quality of heart failure care in minority communities: a randomized trial. *Ann Intern Med.* Vol. 145, No. 4, pp. 273-283.

Smith, G.D.; Hart, C.; Blane, D.; Gillis, C. & Hawthorne, V. (1997). Lifetime socioeconomic position and mortality: prospective observational study. *Br Med J.* Vol. 314, No. 7080, pp. 547.

Smith, G.D; Hart, C.; Blane, D. & Hole, D. (1998). Adverse socioeconomic conditions in childhood and cause specific adult mortality: prospective observational study. *Br Med J.* Vol. 316, No. 7145, pp.1631.

Stanfeld, S.A. (2006). Social support and social cohesion. In, *Social Determinants of Health, Second Edition.* Marmot M and Wilkinson RG, Eds. Oxford University Press, Oxford, UK.

Statistics Canada (1997). National Population Health Survey (NPHS) Asthma Supplement 1996/97. *Health Canada.* Accessed from
<http://www.phac-aspc.gc.ca/publicat/pma-pca00/pdf/asthma00e.pdf>

Stone E.G.; Morton, S.C. &, Hulscher, M.E., et al. (2002) Interventions that increase use of adult immunization and cancer screening services: a meta-analysis. *Ann Intern Med.* Vol. 136, No. 99, pp. 641-651.

U.S. Department of Health and Human Services. (2011). HHS Action Plan to reduce Racial and Ethnic Health Disparities. *U.S. Department of Health and Human Services.* Washington, D.C., USA.

UNDP. (2011). Millennium Development Goals: Where do we stand? United Nations Development Programme, 09-11-2011, Available from,

<http://www.beta.undp.org/undp/en/home/mdgoverview/mdg_goals/mdg1/ Where_do_we_stand.html>

UNESCO. (1998). Statement of Commitment for Action to Eradicate Poverty Adopted by Administrative Committee on Coordination. *United Nations Educational Scientific and Cultural* Organization, 09-11-2011, Available from:
<http://www.unesco.org/most/acc4pov.htm: Oxford University Press, 2006.

United Nations Committee on Social, Economic and Cultural Rights. (2001). Poverty: the Human Rights Approach. UNESCO, 09-11-2011, Available from:
http://www.unesco.org/new/en/social-and-human-sciences/themes/human-rights/poverty-eradication>.

US Department of Health and Human Services. (2011). HHS Action Plan to Reduce Racial and Ethnic Health Disparities: A Nation Free of Disparities in Health and Health Care. *US Department of Health and Human Services.* Available at:
<http://minorityhealth.hhs.gov/npa/files/Plans/HHS/HHS_Plan_complete.pdf>

Valentine, N.; Orielle, S.; Irwin, S.; Nolen, L. & Prasad, A. (2008). Health Equity at the Country Level: Building Capacities and Momentum for Action. *World Health Organization.* 09-11-2011, Available at:
<http://www.who.int/social_determinants/media/sdhe_csw_final_report.pdf>

Van Ryn, M. &, Burke, J. (2000). The effect of patient race and socio-economic status on physicians' perceptions of patients. *Soc Sci Med.* 2000; Vol. 50, No. 6, pp. 813-828.

Vargas Bustamante, A. & Chen, J. (2011) Physicians cite hurdles ranging from lack of coverage to poor communication in providing high quality care to Latinos. *Health Affairs.* Vol. 30, No. 10, pp. 1921-1929.

Walks, R.A. & Bourne, L.S. (2006). Ghettos in Canada's cities? Racial segregation, ethnic enclaves and poverty concentration in Canadian urban areas. *The Canadian Geographer.* Vol. 50, No. 3, pp. 273–29.

Warren, A.G.; Londono, G.E.; Wessel, L.A. &, Warren R.D. (2006). Breaking down barriers to breast and cervical cancer screening: a university-based prevention program for Latinas. *J Health Care Poor Underserved.* Vol. 17, No. 3, pp. 512-521.

Weiss, B.D.; Blanchard, J.S.; McGee, D.L. & Hart, G. (1994). Illiteracy among Medicaid Recipients and its Relationship to Health Care Costs. *J Health Care for the Poor and Underserved.* Vol. 5, No. 2, pp. 99-111.

Woolf, K. & Dacre, J. (2011). Reducing bias in decision making improves care and influences medical student education. *Medical Education.* Vol. 45, pp. 762-764.

Woolf, S.H. (2007). Future health consequences of the current decline in US household income. *JAMA.* Vol. 298, No. 16, pp. 1931-3.

Woolf, S.H.; Johnson, R.E. & Geiger, H.J. (2006) The rising prevalence of severe poverty in America: a growing threat to public health. *Am J Prev Med* Vol. 31, No. 4, pp.332-41.

World Bank (2000). Poverty and Inequality Analysis, In: *The World Bank: Poverty Reduction & Equity,* 09-11-2011, Available from: <http://go.worldbank.org/VFPEGF7FU0>

World Health Organization Commission on the Social Determinants of Health. (2008) Closing the gap in a generation: Health equity through action on the social determinants of health. 09-11-2011.Available at

<http://www.who.int/social_determinants/thecommission/finalreport/en/index
.html>
World Health Organization. (2011). CLOSING THE GAP: Policy into Practice on Social
    Determinants of Health: Discussion Paper. *World Conference on Social Determinants
    of Health*.
Yaggy, S.D.; Michener, J.L., & Yaggy, D. et al. (2006). Just for Us: an academic medical
    center-community partnership to maintain the health of a frail low-income senior
    population. *Gerontologist*. 2006; Vol. 46, No. 2, pp. 271-276.
Ziglio, E.; Barberosa, R.; Charpak, Y. & Turner, S. (2003). Health Systems Confront Poverty.
    World Health Organization, Copenhagen: World Health Organization, 2003.

Primary Care and Non-Physician Clinicians

James F. Cawley[1], Roderick S. Hooker[2] and Diana Crowley[3]
[1]Department of Prevention and Community Health
[2]School of Public Health and Health Services
[3]School of Medicine and Health Sciences
The George Washington University
USA

1. Introduction

The entry point for most people into any healthcare system is primary care. Not surprisingly, primary care–oriented disorders make up the vast majority of all medical conditions seen by healthcare providers. Starfield (1994) pointed out that countries whose health systems are oriented toward primary care achieve better health levels, higher satisfaction with health services among their populations, and lower expenditures in the overall delivery of health care. The American system relies heavily on both physicians as well as nonphysician clinicians to deliver primary care. In the US this cadre of providers includes doctors, PAs and nurse practitioners (NPs).

A substantial amount of research documents that physician assistants (PAs) and NPs are ideally suited and well qualified to deliver primary care services. PAs are trained to diagnose and treat most general medical conditions and a substantial proportion of clinical PAs work in the primary care disciplines. In terms of medical specialties, American primary care is defined as family medicine, general internal medicine, general pediatrics, and sometimes obstetrics and gynecology (as also identified as *women's health*).

Since 1997 the United States has witnessed a decline in primary care physicians (Bodenheimer 2009). This decreasing trend of graduating medical students entering the primary care field has opened more opportunities for PAs and NPs. The education foundation of PAs is primary care and as such they continue to grow as an appealing complement for providing primary care services. This trend will remain as medical school becomes increasingly more expensive; students facing debt pressures select specialty areas because a primary care physician's salary is substanti ally less than that of a specialist such as a surgeon. As the primary care physicians continue to be overworked and highly sought out by patients, the field requires a significant boost in support and supply. We argue on the basis of simple supply and demand the job outlook for PAs in primary care will continue for a few decades.

To most clinicians, the term *primary care* is synonymous with ambulatory care because less than 0.5% of all conditions seen in primary care result in hospitalization. In many countries, general medicine (also known as general practice) serves as the entry point to the health system. Countries with well-established primary care systems have doctors serving as "gatekeepers," meaning that patients do not visit specialists, nor are they admitted to hospitals without being referred by general practice doctors. To some, "gatekeeping" represents a negative element of healthcare delivery systems because patients may be denied needed care. The practice, however, is associated with the avoidance of unnecessary procedures and overtreatment, thus facilitating the appropriate distribution and utilization of limited resources (Franks et al, 1992). In the United States, people can access some specialists directly (e.g. dermatology), which may lead to increased cost and fragmentation of services.

The major focus of medical education for PAs, doctors, and most nurse practitioner (NP) is primary care. Curricula for the would-be primary care clinician are organized so that the graduate can manage most medical conditions in a typical community with a normal population distribution. In many instances, primary care forms the foundation on which other areas of medicine rest. The student entering medicine learns the principles and practice of general medicine. These principles are often incorporated within other specialties, and in turn, specialties develop principles that are adopted in primary care. To understand this crucial role, which PAs and NPs have increasingly helped to define, we first define *primary care*.

2. Primary care defined

Primary care is the provision of integrated, accessible healthcare services by clinicians who are responsible for meeting most personal healthcare needs, developing sustained partnerships with patients, and practicing in the context of family and community. Definitions of primary care typically focus on the type or level of health services such as preventive, diagnostic, and therapeutic services; health education and counseling; and minor surgery, although it is possible for specialists to provide primary care. For example, a cardiologist who offers advanced specialized care for myocardial conditions will also provide health education and preventive counseling.

The most commonly accepted definition of primary care is medical care services that are characterized by the following attributes:

- first-contact care
- longitudinality
- coordination
- comprehensiveness (Starfield, 1993)

Primary health care providers are considered to be the gatekeepers of medicine. In an ideal primary health care system, patients would first have contact with their provider before seeking specialty services. This *first-contact care* is essential for the physician to perform an initial assessment and how to best treat or direct the patient' care. Because there are constraints on the American system of access to care, alternatives to primary care occur. Overflow in US emergency rooms is partly attributed to the fact that the patient cannot access this first step in medical care services.

Another important attribute to holistic primary care service is *longitudinality*, or care provided continually for the patient regardless of the patient's state of health. Annual physicals are an example of this attribute, where primary health care providers can monitor patients over time (Starfield 1979). Longitudinal care not only allows for the primary health care provider to analyze improvements and/or deficiencies in patient health, but also serves as a means for provider and patient to build strong rapport through these annual exams.

Coordination builds off the first attribute in that it utilizes the initial findings to then refer the patient to a trusted partner of the desired service. The primary health care provider must be knowledgeable of the available resources in order to successfully coordinate with the partnering provider and patient. Seamless integration of referring patients and working with specialty providers will lead to a successful collaboration in assessing the needs of the patient (Starfield 1979). Working together in this manner overlaps with the last attribute, comprehensiveness.

Comprehensiveness is difficult to achieve, but necessary to strive for in order to provide the best care for the patient. The primary health care provider is not simply a gatekeeper, but essentially a jack-of-all-trades. As each patient presents health-specific issues, the provider will serve as an educational resource, a prevention advocate, a supporter for positive change in healthy behavior and as a trusted clinician at any one point in time. Recognition of the problem is crucial in both coordinating with other providers and ensuring a complete standard of care (Starfield, 1979).

These four attributes (first-contact, longitudinality, coordination, comprehensiveness) also serve as measurement tools when assessing the quality of primary care service provided. Detractors to the quality of care can often be attributed to inaccessibility, both perceived and actual inaccessibility, as well as poor coordination with other providers (Starfield 2005). Poor coordination can often lead to mistrust in the primary care provider, diminishing the likelihood of longitudinality and thus an incomprehensive level of care.

Primary care is distinguished from two other classifications of healthcare delivery: secondary and tertiary care. *Secondary care* is usually thought of as short-term service delivery, infrequent consultation from a specialist, or surgical or other advanced interventions that primary care clinicians are not equipped to provide (Shi & Singh, 2008). This type of care includes hospitalization, routine surgery, specialty consultation, and rehabilitation. *Tertiary care* is regarded as the provision of care for complex conditions and usually involves an institution with advanced technology and specialty and subspecialty services (Hooker 2008). Examples include organ transplants, burn centers, cardiothoracic surgery centers, and advanced trauma centers.

The World Health Organization (WHO) Meeting on Primary Care, Family Medicine/General Practice in Barcelona, Spain, in 2002 proposed a definition of *primary care*: "Primary care refers to a span or an assembly of first-contact healthcare services directly accessible to the public." Accessibility is an important aspect of primary care to consider because it directly relates to the health outcome of the patient and cost of care. Researchers at the 2003 WHO conference believe an increased supply of primary care physicians would lead to a healthier population (Starfield 2005). This would help correct for the uneven distribution of physician specialty fields, thus increasing accessibility and decreasing health care cost.

Essentially, primary care strives to be as accessible as possible to the community it serves. This emphasis on accessibility has led to the growth of community-oriented primary care

(COPC). COPC serves as the bridge between clinical medicine and public health. COPC is no stranger to the field of primary care, with its roots dating back to the 1940s, but due to the attention regarding increased health outcomes related to COPC systems, primary care strives to adopt this focus (Gofin 2005). This community-based effort encompasses the four attributes of primary care: first-contact care, longitudinality, coordination and comprehensiveness.

Primary care (as opposed to primary *health* care) has gained increased attention since the new century and raised several questions. For example, how does it fit into the healthcare delivery system? Is it the same as primary health care? What strategies should be used to link primary care with other levels of care? What are the implications of developments in technology for primary care functions and professionals? These are some of the issues many countries in the WHO European Region are facing when trying to develop primary care as part of the overall healthcare system.

The participants of the 2002 WHO conference in Barcelona concluded that primary care is part of the provision of healthcare services and has to be looked at in the context of the overall services, not in isolation. In light of the confusion about commonly used terms—notably *primary healthcare, primary care, primary medical care, general practice,* and *family medicine*—the consensus was that a clear distinction between *primary health care* (as presented in the Declaration of Alma-Ata in 1978) and *primary care* (which refers to local level healthcare services) was necessary. More work in this area will emerge before the end of this decade.

3. Primary care ecology

Human medical ecology may be defined as the study of relationships between people and the medical care system. One of the most famous and revealing studies of primary care was conducted by Kerr White and colleagues, titled "The Ecology of Medical Care" (White, Williams, & Greenberg, 1961). They drew a portrait of people, illness, and medical care that assumed a typical population of 1,000 citizens in an average month. The results were drawn from 1,000 non-institutionalized adults; 750 were symptomatic for some illness each month, 250 received care from doctors in the office setting, 9 were hospitalized, 5 were referred to a specialist, and no more than 1 was admitted to a tertiary medical center or hospital. The authors were trying to make the point that health policies in the United States tended to overemphasize hospital-based care and that the common problems that people had most of the time were relegated to the underfunded, underappreciated system of primary care.

Forty years later, the study was replicated with expanded and updated data (Green, 2001). The results were remarkably similar. In an average month, again using 1,000 men, women, and children in the United States, about 800 were symptomatic, 327 considered seeking medical care, 217 visited a doctor, 65 visited a provider of complementary and alternative medicine, 21 visited a hospital outpatient clinic, 14 received care in their home, 8 were hospitalized, and no more than 1 was hospitalized in an academic medical center. These findings indicate the relative occurrence and severity of health problems in the U.S. population and the choices that persons make regarding the medical care system. The 2001 findings reaffirm the portrait of a health system that has a well-funded, high-technology tertiary health component that serves only a fraction of the ill population that needs a more extensive and better supported system of primary care (Green, 2001).

4. Effectiveness

Effectiveness of primary care delivery depends, at least in part, on using the correct mix of personnel. Starfield (1994) showed that the division of labor and economy of scale maximizes the clinical capabilities of healthcare professionals. In primary care practice, it is neither necessary nor particularly efficient for each patient to be seen by a physician. Since PAs are, by definition, physician-supervised clinicians, the very nature of their clinical role is to work with doctors in collaborative provider teams. To be effective, the PA needs to provide quality care to similar patients for similar diagnoses that result in outcomes comparable to those of a doctor. Several studies have been conducted which compare the care provided by PAs and doctors on quality measures including processes of care and/or patient outcomes for specific diagnoses.

5. The primary care workforce in the US

The primary care workforce in the United States consists of primary care physicians, nurse practitioners (NPs), and physician assistants (PAs). Are PAs and NPs the future of primary care practice? Given the concurrent trends of increasing calls to strengthen the primary care workforce, declining physician attraction to primary care residency training, and increasing reliance on PAs and NPs to deliver primary care services, there is evidence to support this assertion. A recent data report from the National Center for Health Statistics provides validation of this latter trend using information from hospital outpatient departments. The data brief (Hing, 2011) reveals that hospital outpatient department visits handled by PAs and NPs (and other advanced practice nurses [APN}) increased from 10% in 2000 and 2001 to 15% in 2008 and 2009. This suggests a wider degree of utilization of PAs and NPs, particularly in settings where a good deal of primary care services are delivered. PA and NP involvement in providing services varied by location, with these providers handling 36% of visits in nonmetropolitan centers versus only 6% of visits in urban hospitals. Also, the size of the hospital outpatient department was related to whether patients were seen exclusively by a PA or NP, with 24% of such visits in hospitals with fewer than 200 beds, and only 10% in facilities with 400 or more beds. PAs and NPs also delivered care more often in clinics associated with nonteaching hospitals and handled a higher percentage of Medicaid, CHIP, or uninsured patients, as well as younger patients. These data suggest that PAs and NPs are used to a greater degree in smaller facilities located in non-urban areas to serve populations that may be otherwise medically underserved, trends that are consistent with the original policy intentions of their creators. The NCHS report confirms that PAs and NPs "continue to provide a critical health care function" by administering care in communities that are prone to physician shortages, including in rural, small, and nonteaching hospitals (Hing, 2011).

The data brief results also provide a small window into the content of care delivered by PAs and NPs, an area in which the literature is sparse. PAs and NPs saw a higher percentage of visits where a new problem was the major reason for the visit (22%) compared with visits for a chronic condition (11%) or pre/postsurgery care (6%). Of particular interest to some is the finding that PAs and NPs saw a higher percentage of preventive care visits (17%) compared with visits for a routine chronic condition or pre/postsurgical care. It has long been speculated that PAs and NPs certainly have the potential to provide care that is more prevention-oriented than physician care, and it appears that they may be fulfilling this potential. Further delineation of this trend is warranted. Practicing preventive medicine to a greater degree may offer even further justification not only for the widespread utilization of PAs and NPs in primary care but also for policy changes leading to greater levels of reimbursement for preventive services by third-party health payors.

While the absolute number of primary care physicians, nurse practitioners and physician assistants is expected to rise in the coming years, these changes are not expected to be sufficient to meet the demands of an aging population, changes in service use, and trends connected with a major expansion of insurance coverage. The best estimates of the primary care provider supply continue to indicate that there are significant shortages. According to new numbers from the DHHS Agency for Healthcare Quality and Research, as of 2009, only about one-third of the Nation's 625,000 practicing physicians, or about 208,000 providers, work in primary care (AHRQ, 2011); and, as of 2010, about 43.4 percent or 30,300, of the estimated 70,333 PAs in practice, and 52% or 55,626 of the estimated 106,000 NPs in practice, are currently in primary care (AHRQ, 2011). It is believed that these numbers are insufficient to meet current and future demands for primary care services.

Longer term trends point to the establishment of PAs and NPs as the principal front-line providers of primary care services with physicians assuming more managerial and executive functions as well as a greater focus on inpatient specialty practice. A former Deputy Dean and Professor of Medicine at Yale School of Medicine recently observed that "in the decades ahead, it is likely that the main role of the generalist physician will be to supervise those providing primary care and to personally care for patients with complex illnesses who are hospitalized, an idea already well established as the hospitalist movement." He adds further that "the challenge will be to successfully integrate a new primary care system that relies more heavily on nurses and PAs with specialty-based medicine, hopefully through health care reform and the help of a universal electronic medical record" (Gifford, 2011). When it comes to primary care, clearly PAs and NPs are the health care providers who's time has come and in the future will only increase in utilization and influence.

NPs and PAs are health professions begun in the U.S. in the 1960s in response to a shortage and uneven distribution of physicians. They are licensed in all States, but there is considerable variation in the laws governing their scope of practice. They play important roles in many health care fields including primary care.

The Centers for Medicare & Medicaid Services maintains the National Provider Identifier (NPI) dataset, which listed 93,000 practicing NPs and 63,000 practicing PAs in 2009. While this estimate represents approximately 10,000 fewer practicing PAs than projected by the American Academy of Physician Assistants (AAPA), it represents approximately 10,000 more NPs than most other recent estimates. Unfortunately, there is no consistent and comprehensive data source for NPs, which hampers understanding of how many are clinically active, what specialties they practice, and in what settings. It is estimated that in 2011, there are roughly 80,00 PAs in active clinical practice with 34% in primary care specialties.

To further inform policy discussions around the U.S. primary care workforce, the Agency for Healthcare Research and Quality's (AHRQ) Center for Primary Care, Prevention, and Clinical Partnerships identified the number of primary care providers in 2010: *The Number of Practicing Primary Care Physicians in the U.S.*, which reports that, of the 624,434 physicians in the United States who spend the majority of their time in direct patient care, slightly less than one-third are specialists in primary care.

6. The future of primary care

In the US, states with a higher proportion of primary care physicians to population consistently report a population with healthier outcomes (Starfield 2005). Factors including inaccessibility, cost, changing health care system and decrease supply of primary care physicians most likely contribute to decreasing ratios of primary care providers to population. PAs and NPs will play an integral role as the physician specialty gap continues to widen.

This relationship between primary care physician supply and health of the associated population is seen outside of the US as well. Studies similar to the one in the US was replicated in England and produced similar results, revealing an overall reduced mortality rate for areas with high ratios of primary care physicians. Similar results have been seen on a global scale, highlighting the healthcare gap between rural and urban areas.

7. Global growth of nonphysicians

The global expansion of physician assistants (PAs) and nurse practitioners (NPs) is a medical workforce trend that began in the 1970s but did not blossom until the turn of the century. As of 2012, at least 10 countries are in various stages of integrating PA and or NP-like medical care providers who function under the broad supervision of a doctor. Countries that have documented their development include Australia, Canada, England, the Netherlands, Scotland, South Africa, and Germany. Several of these these countries have American-trained PAs working as expatriates and most have developed educational programs aimed at producing healthcare providers functioning as assistants to licensed physicians. Other countries with PAs and NPs, but less known in their development, include Ghana, Liberia, and India. Each country has made the PA a distinct entity within their health systems, each with their own cultural and educational influences shaping their roles. The PAs and NPs have common denominators:

They are semiautonomous clinicians who function under the supervision of a doctor, complementing their capacities to deliver healthcare services. Historical patterns suggest that the development and evolution of PAs and NPs in health systems follow similar steps, suggesting there are useful lessons learned in the utilization of nonphysician providers that may prove useful in improving the delivery of primary care services (Cawley and Hooker, 2003). Shortages of doctors, especially in rural areas and in primary care practice; rising healthcare costs; and increases in physician specialization have resulted in a number of countries looking to nonphysician providers (PAs and NPs) as augmenting forces to medical workforce problems. For instance, England faces a challenge as a result of meeting the European Union directive to reduce the number of hours house officers are permitted to work. Canada not only has doctor shortages, but also must continue to cope with healthcare access problems for many of its citizens, including those in rural areas. The Netherlands must meet rising numbers of older patients with chronic disease, multiple co-morbidities, and escalating costs of health care. These countries and others have turned their interests to developing a U.S.-modeled PA and/or NP practitioner to work closely with the doctor and to improve access to care.

It is evident that primary care is an essential component of any health care system to ensure an appropriate standard of care for all populations. It is also evident that the supply of these health care providers has and will continue to decrease in the upcoming years. Additionally, the burden of increased responsibility for these physicians in recent years contributes to this trend of lacking primary care physicians (Bodenheimer 2009). Several questions remain regarding the future of the field. Ultimately, accessibility, the number of providers and the cost of primary care will dictate how primary care is provided in the future.

8. References

Bodenheimer, T. (2009). A lifeline for primary care. *New England Journal of Medicine.* 360, 2693-2696.

Cawley, JF, Hooker, RS. Physician Assistants: Does the US Experience Have Anything to Offer Other Countries? *Journal of Health Services Research and Policy* 2003;8:65-67.

Franks, P., Clancy, C. M., & Nutting, P. A. (1992). Gatekeeping revisited: Protecting patients from overtreatment. *New England Journal of Medicine, 327*(21), 424–429.

Gofin, J. & Gofin, R. (2005). Community-oriented primary care and primary health care. *American Journal of Public Health.* 95(5). 757

Green L.A., et al (2001). The ecology of medical care revisited. *New England Journal of Medicine. 344* (26), 2021-2025.

Gifford, R. The Future of Primary Care. Primary Care Progress, October, 2011. Accessed at: http://primarycareprogress.org/blogs/16/102.

Hing, E., Uddin, S. Physician Assistant and Advanced Practice Nurse Care in Hospital Outpatient Departments: United States, 2008-2009. National Center for Health Statistics, Data Brief, No. 77, November, 2011.

Hooker, R. S., Cipher, D. J., Cawley, J. F., Herrmann, D., & Melson, J. (2008). Emergency medicine services: Interprofessional care trends. *Journal of Interprofessional Care, 22*(2), 167–178.

Primary Care Workforce Facts and Stats: Overview. AHRQ Publication No. 12-P001-1-EF, October 2011. Agency for Health Care Policy and Research, Rockville, MD. http://www.ahrq.gov/research/pcworkforce.htm

Primary Care Workforce Facts and Stats No. 2: The Number of Nurse Practitioners and Physician Assistants Practicing Primary Care in the United States. AHRQ Publication No. 12-P001-3-EF, October 2011. Agency for Health Care Policy and Research, Rockville, MD. http://www.ahrq.gov/research/pcwork2.htm

Shi, L., & Singh, D. A. (2008). *Delivering Health Care in America.* Sudbury, MA: Jones & Bartlett.

Starfield, B. (1994). Is primary care essential? *Lancet. 344* (8930), 1129-1133.

Starfield, B. (1979). Measuring the attainment of primary care. *Journal of Medical Education.* 54, 361-369.

Starfield, B, Shi, L, & Macinko, J. (2005). Contribution of primary care to health systems and health. *The Milbank Quarterly.* 83 (2), 457-502.

White,K.; Williams,T.F.; Greenberg,B. (1961). The ecology of medical care. *New England Journal of Medicine.* 265 885-892.

Section 2

Comprehensiveness of Primary Care

4

Integrating Spirituality into Primary Care

Giancarlo Lucchetti[1,2,3], Alessandra L. Granero Lucchetti[1],
Rodrigo M. Bassi[1], Alejandro Victor Daniel Vera[1,3]
and Mario F. P. Peres[1,3]
1São Paulo Medical Spiritist Association,
2João Evangelista Hospital,
3Federal University of São Paulo,
Brazil

1. Introduction

Spirituality has been associated with medical care for centuries. Hospitals and universities originally were based on religious tenants and grounded by religious temples or societies. Nevertheless, in the early part of the 20th century there was a separation between religion, spirituality and medicine as the emphasis of medicine shifted to a more scientific focus(1).

However, since the 1960´s, epidemiological studies started to show the impact of religiosity and spirituality to the patient health and triggered research on this subject. Religion was seen by many as beneficial and responsible for clinical outcomes, which motivated the creation of the term "Evidence Based Spirituality"(2, 3).

Since then, thousands of articles have been published in scientific databases showing the impact of religiosity/spirituality in mental and physical health(4, 5). Spirituality has been associated with quality of life, better mental health, survival, less hospitalization and better coping (6-8).

In addition, patients believe their doctors should ask about spiritual matters which could improve the doctor-patient relationship. According to recent studies, 99 percent of family physicians believe that religious beliefs can heal, and 75 percent believe that others' prayers can promote healing(9).

Nevertheless, physicians usually are not trained for addressing spiritual beliefs and reported many barriers for that evaluation such as: lack of time, lack of knowledge, lack of training, fear and being not comfortable to address it(10).

Spirituality is defined by Koenig(11) as "a personal search for understanding final questions about life, its meaning, its relationships to sacredness or transcendence that may or may not lead to the development of religious practices or formation of religious communities".

Religiosity(11) is understood as the "extension to which an individual believes, follows, and practices a religion, and can be organizational (church or temple attendance) or non organizational (to pray, to read books, to watch religious programs on television)".

In fact, many arguments support the teaching and practice of these basic spiritual/religious skills to physicians(3, 12, 13):

1.   Religious beliefs and spiritual needs are common among patients, and many patients would like their doctors to address these issues
2.   Religious beliefs influence medical decision making
3.   There is a relationship between spirituality and health.
4.   Supporting a patient's spirituality can enrich the patient-physician relationship.

In this chapter, we aim to investigate the role of spirituality and religiosity in primary care, reviewing the following topics (Box 1).

1.   scientific evidence of the relation between spirituality and health
2.   primary care patients and physicians' opinions
3.   reasons for addressing
4.   barriers
5.   how to address spiritual issues in clinical practice
6.   religious struggle
7.   ethical issues
8.   the role of primary care physician.

Box 1. Topics addressed by this chapter

2. Scientific evidence of the relation between spirituality and health

There is a huge amount of evidence regarding the impact of spirituality/religiousness in health.

For instance, a search conducted in the beginning of 2011 showed that 4.42 articles per day were published on Pubmed concerning spirituality or religion. Furthermore, the most important and high quality journals in the World have been publishing these articles such as New England Journal of Medicine(14), The Journal of the American Medical Association (15) and Lancet (9).

Most American Universities have departments dealing with this kind of issue such as "The George Washington Institute for Spirituality and Health from George Washington University", "Center for Spirituality, theology and health from Duke UNiversity" and Center for the study of Health, Religion and Spirituality from Indiana State University among others. In addition, most American medical schools have spirituality courses in their curriculum (16).

In "Handbook of Religion and Health"(11, 17), authors analyzed all articles published in scientific databases before the year 2000. From those, more than 700 studies examined the relation between religion, well-being, and mental health. They found that religious beliefs and practices were associated with significantly less depression and faster recovery from depression (60 of 93 studies), lower suicide rates (57 of 68), less anxiety (35 of 69), and less substance abuse (98 of 120). They were also associated with greater well-being, hope, and optimism (91 of 114), more purpose and meaning in life (15 of 16), greater marital satisfaction and stability (35 of 38) and higher social support (19 of 20).

A summary of the research on physical health outcomes(11, 17) found that religious beliefs and activities have been associated with better immune function (5 of 5 studies); lower death rates from cancer (5 of 7); less heart disease or better cardiac outcomes (7 of 11); lower blood pressure (14 of 23); lower cholesterol (3 of 3): and better health behaviors (23 of 25, less cigarette smoking; 3 of 5, more exercise; 2 of 2, better sleep).

Some other studies have studied the relation between spirituality and religiousness (S/R) and survival. Three meta-analysis(5, 18, 19) found that patients with higher levels of spiritual/religious beliefs have a lower mortality (varying from a 18 to 25% decrease) and a recent study(7) found that S/R plays a considerable role in mortality rate reductions, comparable to fruit and vegetable consumption and statin therapy.

Recently, some studies have been addressing the impact of a spiritual intervention for treatment of some conditions such as anxiety(20), depression(21),cancer(22), including others.

3. Primary care patients and physicians' opinions

According to recent surveys, most patients want their doctors to ask about their religious and/or spiritual beliefs.

McCord et al.(23) evaluated 921 patients and found that 83% of respondents wanted physicians to ask about spiritual beliefs. The most acceptable scenarios for spiritual discussion were life-threatening illnesses (77%), serious medical conditions (74%) and loss of loved ones (70%). Among those who wanted to discuss spirituality, the most important reason for discussion was desire for physician-patient understanding (87%). Patients believed that information concerning their spiritual beliefs would affect physicians' ability to encourage realistic hope (67%), give medical advice (66%), and change medical treatment (62%).

Ehman et al.(24) also evaluated patient acceptance of including a spiritual beliefs question in the medical history of ambulatory outpatients. They found that forty-five percent of patients believe religious beliefs would influence their medical decisions if they become gravely ill. Further, ninety-four percent of individuals agreed that physicians should ask them whether they have such beliefs if they become gravely ill. Altogether, two thirds of the respondents indicated that they would welcome a spirituality question in a medical history, whereas 16% reported that they would not. Only 15% of the study group recalled having been asked whether spiritual or religious beliefs would influence their medical decisions.

In other countries, these results are similar. Lucchetti et al.(6) evaluated rehabilitation Brazilian patients and found that more than 87% of patients wanted their physicians to ask about their religious beliefs. Nevertheless, only 8.7% recalled have been asked about their religion by their doctors.

Primary care physicians have been asked several times about these issues. Luckhaupt et al.(25) evaluated the opinions of primary care residents and found that 46% felt they should play a role in patients' spiritual or religious lives, especially when the gravity of patient's condition increased.

In 2003, Monroe et al.(26) evaluated primary care physicians and found that 84.5% of them thought they should be aware of patients' spirituality. However, most would not ask about spiritual issues unless a patient was dying. They also found that family practitioners were more likely to take a spiritual history than general internists.

Another study conducted by Ellis et al.(27) showed that 96% of 231 family physicians interviewed considered spiritual well-being an important health component, 86% supported referral of hospitalized patients with spiritual questions to chaplains, and 58% believed physicians should address patients' spiritual concerns. According to the authors, fear of dying was the spiritual issue most commonly discussed, and less than 20% of physicians reported discussing other spiritual topics in more than 10% of patient encounters.

4. Reasons for addressing

Many reasons are pointed up for addressing spirituality in clinical practice. Table 1 shows the most common reasons pointed and their explanation.

In addition, the JCAHO(13) (Joint Commission on Accreditation of Healthcare Organizations) requires that a spiritual history be taken and documented on every patient admitted to a hospital, nursing home or home health care agency.

Reasons for addressing	Explanation (According to recent surveys)
Religious beliefs and spiritual needs are common among patients	90-99% of patients believe in God and 70% are church/temple members(3, 13)
Many patients would like their doctors to address these issues	More than 80% of patients want physicians to ask about spiritual beliefs and more than 94% if they become very ill(23, 24)
Religious beliefs influence medical decision making	Near half of the patients believe religious beliefs would influence their medical decisions if they become gravely ill. In addition, religious beliefs could influence diet, blood transfusion, use of contraceptive methods, including others(13, 24).
Many patients depend on religion to cope	More than 80-90% of the population usually turn to religion in order to cope with stressful events(13, 28)
Religious/spiritual beliefs can impact mental and physical health	Spirituality and religiousness have relation to almost every aspect of the human being. These evidences were extensively discussed earlier in this chapter.(11)
Supporting a patient's spirituality can enrich the patient-physician relationship.	66 to 81% would have greater trust in their physician if he asked about their religious beliefs, including an improvement of patient-physician relationship(13)
Religious involvement may affect the kind of support and care patients receive in the community	Religious organizations could play a role in early disease prevention (education), early disease detection (screening) and provision of health care (trained volunteerings).(13)

Table 1. Reasons for addressing spiritual issues

5. Barriers

Many barriers are pointed up by health professionals for not including spirituality and religiousness issues in their daily routine.

Ellis et al.(27) found in primary care physicians that the most common barriers were: lack of time (71%), inadequate training for taking spiritual histories (59%), and difficulty identifying patients who want to discuss spiritual issues (56%).

The same author(29) also divided the barriers in four parts: Physician Barriers, Mutual Physician–Patient Barriers, Physician-Perceived Patient Barriers and Situational Barriers (Table 2).

Barriers	Types of Barriers
Physician Barriers	Lack of comfort or training Lack of spiritual awareness or inclination Fear of inappropriately influencing patients
Mutual Physician–Patient Barriers	Discomfort with initiating discussions Lack of concordance between physician and patient spiritual or cultural positions No common "spiritual language"
Physician-Perceived Patient Barriers	Fear that it's wrong to ask doctor spiritual questions Belief that spiritual views are private Perception of physician time pressure
Situational Barriers	Time Setting (examination room) Lack of continuity or managed care

Table 2. Most common barriers for incorporating spirituality in clinical practice(29).

A recent survey evaluated the barriers pointed up by medical teachers from a Brazilian medical school regarding integrating spirituality in clinical practice and found that the most prevalent barriers cited by medical teachers were: lack of time (11.3%), lack of knowledge (9.3%), lack of training (9.3%), fear (9.3%) and being not comfortable to address it (5.6%).

6. How to address spiritual issues in clinical practice

Health professionals experience difficulties assessing this issue in clinical practice(26). In order to facilitate the addressing of spirituality in clinical practice, several authors have created instruments to obtain a spiritual history (30-32).

Anandarajah et al. suggested that a spiritual assessment should include "determination of spiritual needs and resources, evaluation of the impact of beliefs on medical outcomes and decisions, discovery of barriers to using spiritual resources and encouragement of healthy spiritual practices"(31).

According to the Joint Commission on Accreditation of Healthcare Organizations JCAHO(33), practitioners should conduct an initial, brief spiritual assessment with clients in many settings, including hospitals and behavioral health organizations providing addiction services. The same framework, however, is used in all settings. At minimum, the brief assessment should include an exploration of three areas: (1) denomination or faith tradition, (2) significant spiritual beliefs, and (3) important spiritual practices.

Table 3 shows some important instruments to facilitate spirituality addressing in clinical practice by primary care physicians.

Instrument	Opinion
SPIRITual History(34)	This instrument is very broad, evaluating key questions such as medical practices not allowed and terminal events. Nevertheless, it takes a relatively long time to apply which can hamper its use in certain settings, especially those involving 15 to 20 minutes primary care (general practitioner) consultations.
FICA (30)	Easy to remember and to apply, and was well suited for those physicians that want to address patients' spirituality but do not have enough time for a consultation. It covers the social aspect as well as treatment action. It also constitutes a good instrument for those beginning in this field and with little training.
HOPE (31)	Good instrument that is easy to remember and which addresses important questions such as medical practices not allowed and personal spirituality
FACT – Spiritual history tool (35)	a straight-forward instrument which is quick to apply, has a treatment plan, and includes a question about coping
CSI-MEMO Spiritual History (32)	Easy to remember, easy to use, fast to apply, and address important questions such as coping (comfort), the negative side of religion (stress) and the influence of spiritual beliefs on medical decisions
Spiritual history of the American College of Physicians (36)	Fast to apply and easy to address. Nevertheless, some important questions pertaining to palliative care such as medical practices not allowed due to religion and terminal events, are not included.

Table 3. Some instruments to facilitate spirituality addressing in clinical practice by primary care physicians.

7. Religious/spiritual struggles

Religious/spiritual struggles refer to expressions of conflict, question, doubt, and tension about matters of faith, God, and religious relationships that occur as an individual attempts to conserve or transform a spirituality that has been threatened or harmed (37). Spiritual struggles can be triggered by a variety of stressors. For example, a single unexpected event, such as the untimely loss of a loved one, may overtax the orientation system and trigger a spiritual struggle.

It is important for the primary care physician to differ the religious coping (positive) from the religious struggle (negative) because the first has positive outcomes on patient's health. Nevertheless, the later has extremely negative impacts.

In 2001, Pargament et al.(38) evaluated 596 patients aged 55 years or older and found that higher religious struggle scores at baseline were predictive of greater risk of mortality (risk ratio [RR]: 1.06) during a two-year follow-up.

McConnell et al.(39) investigated the relationship between spiritual struggles and various types of psychopathology symptoms in individuals who had and had not suffered from a recent illness. The authors found that negative religious coping was significantly linked to various forms of psychopathology, including anxiety, phobic anxiety, depression, paranoid ideation, obsessive–compulsiveness, and somatization, after controlling for demographic and religious variables.

Ai et al.(40) examined spiritual struggle related to plasma interleukin-6 (IL-6) in 235 adult patients undergoing cardiac surgery and showed that spiritual struggle (p = .011) were associated with excess plasma IL-6, even after controlling for medical correlates.

8. Ethical issues

Many ethical issues emerged with the incorporation of spirituality in patient care. According to Daaleman (41), "the ethical challenge of intersecting patient and physician spiritualities lies in how both negotiate these movements across health and illness".

The most common ethical issues regarding spirituality, religion and health are (for a deeper reading, see the following references) (23, 42):

- Respect for patients' opinion: Autonomy requires that physicians respect the decisions of competent patients, which are often based on religious and spiritual beliefs
- Not impose physicians' religion: Nonmaleficence ("do no harm") requires that physicians not proselytize.
- End-of-life care and decisions: some end-of-life care decisions as well as life-support decisions were influenced by religious traditions(43).
- Contraception and abortion: Most religions have taken strong positions on abortion and ethical issues are very common on these situations.
- Acceptance of hemocomponents and hemoderivatives: Some religious traditions such as Jehovah's Witnesses refuses to accept hemoderivatives essentially based on the Bible(44).

- Praying with the patient: physicians should not impose their religious beliefs on patients nor initiate prayer without knowledge of the patient's religious background and likely appreciation of such activity(15).

Finally, according to Curlin et al.(45) "Physicians who engage patients in discourse regarding religion should do so in an ethic of friendship, marked by wisdom, candor, and respect. Whether a particular conversation is ethical will depend on the character of those involved and the context of their engagement."

9. The role of primary care physician

Thousands of studies have been showing that just the biological model is not enough for treating the whole patient(46).

According to the World Health Organization (WHO): "Health is a state of complete physical, mental and social well-being and not merely the absence of disease or infirmity" (47).

The WHO definition has been submitted to revision at the end of last decade, under the impulse of Dr Halfdan Mahler, WHO Director-general at that time. The executive board submitted a new definition of health including the spiritual dimension of health in the following way "Health is a state of complete physical, mental, social and spiritual well-being and not merely the absence of disease or infirmity." This modified WHO health definition was to be presented to the 1st World Assembly of Health in 1998 as it requested a revision of the WHO Constitution. Finally, this proposal slipped away from endorsement and has not yet been brought back on the agenda(47). Although not approved yet, this definition is widely use in this new paradigm of integrative medicine.

Integrative medicine represents a higher-order system of systems of care that emphasizes wellness and healing of the entire person (bio-psycho-socio-spiritual dimensions) as primary goals, drawing on both conventional and CAM approaches in the context of a supportive and effective physician-patient relationship(46).

The aims of primary care are to provide the patient with a broad spectrum of care, both preventive and curative, over a period of time and to coordinate all of the care the patient receives(48). In other words, primary care physicians have the responsibility of providing the best care available for their patients and, if their patients have a spiritual issue they need to know how to act. Further, most available studies dealing with this issue have been conducted in primary care settings and by primary care researchers (49).

According to Walter Larimore(50): "Just as 'obstetrics is just too important to be left to obstetricians' I believe the practice of basic spiritual skills is just too important to be left solely to pastoral professionals." The authors of this chapter share this view.

10. Conclusion

In conclusion, spirituality and its interface with medicine have been extensively discussed and considered by health professionals, including those responsible for primary care.

The patient care, previously limited only to the biology dimension, is now being expanded to other dimensions (social, psychological, spiritual) in a more integrative and complex view.

Health professionals should be aware of the spiritual beliefs/needs of their patients in order to treat them as fully as possible.

11. References

[1] Koenig HG. Religion and medicine I: historical background and reasons for separation. International Journal of Psychiatry in Medicine. 2000;30(4):385-98.

[2] Saad M, Masiero D, Battistella LR. Espiritualidade baseada em evidências (Evidence-based Spirituality). Acta Fisiátrica. 2001;8(1):18-23.

[3] Lucchetti G, Granero AL, Bassi RM, Latorraca R, Nacif S. Espiritualidade na prática clínica: o que o clínico deve saber. Rev Bras Clin Med. 2010;8(2):154-8.

[4] Seybold KS, Hill PC. The role of religion and spirituality in mental and physical health. Current Directions in Psychological Science. 2001;10(1):21-4.

[5] Powell LH, Shahabi L, Thoresen CE. Religion and spirituality: Linkages to physical health. American Psychologist. 2003;58(1):36-52.

[6] Lucchetti G, Lucchetti AGL, Badan-Neto AM, Peres PT, Peres MFP, Moreira-Almeida A, et al. Religiousness Affects Mental Health, Pain and Quality of Life in Older People in an Outpatient Rehabilitation Setting. Journal of Rehabilitation Medicine. 2011;43(4):316-22.

[7] Lucchetti G, Lucchetti ALG, Koenig HG. Impact of Spirituality/Religiosity on Mortality: Comparison With Other Health Interventions. EXPLORE: The Journal of Science and Healing. 2011;7(4):234-8.

[8] Miller WR, Thoresen CE. Spirituality, religion, and health: An emerging research field. American Psychologist. 2003;58(1):24-35.

[9] Sloan RP, Bagiella E, Powell T. Religion, spirituality, and medicine. LANCET. 1999;353:664-7.

[10] Mariotti L, Lucchetti G, Dantas M, Banin V, Fumelli F, Padula N. Spirituality and medicine: views and opinions of teachers in a Brazilian medical school. Medical teacher. 2011;33(4):339-40.

[11] Koenig HG, McCullough ME, Larson DB. Handbook of religion and health: Oxford University Press, USA; 2001.

[12] Mills PJ. Spirituality, religiousness, and health: From research to clinical practice. Annals of Behavioral Medicine. 2002;24(1):1-2.

[13] Koenig HG. Spirituality in patient care: why, how, when, and what: Templeton Press; 2007.

[14] Sloan RP, Bagiella E, VandeCreek L, Hover M, Casalone C, Hirsch TJ, et al. Should physicians prescribe religious activities? New England Journal of Medicine. 2000;342(25):1913-6.

[15] Koenig HG. Religion, spirituality, and medicine: Application to clinical practice. JAMA: the journal of the American Medical Association. 2000;284(13):1708.

[16] Fortin AH, Barnett KG. Medical school curricula in spirituality and medicine. JAMA: the journal of the American Medical Association. 2004;291(23):2883.

[17] Koenig HG. Religion, spirituality, and medicine: research findings and implications for clinical practice. Southern Medical Journal. 2004;97(12):1194-200.

[18] Chida Y, Steptoe A, Powell LH. Religiosity/spirituality and mortality. Psychotherapy and psychosomatics. 2009;78(2):81-90.

[19] McCullough ME, Hoyt WT, Larson DB, Koenig HG, Thoresen C. Religious involvement and mortality: A meta-analytic review. Health Psychology. 2000;19(3):211-22.

[20] Koszycki D, Raab K, Aldosary F, Bradwejn J. A multifaith spiritually based intervention for generalized anxiety disorder: a pilot randomized trial. Journal of clinical psychology. 2010;66(4):430-41.

[21] Rajagopal D, Mackenzie E, Bailey C, Lavizzo-Mourey R. The effectiveness of a spiritually-based intervention to alleviate subsyndromal anxiety and minor depression among older adults. Journal of Religion and Health. 2002;41(2):153-66.

[22] Cole B, Pargament K. Re creating your life: a spiritual/psychotherapeutic intervention for people diagnosed with cancer. Psycho Oncology. 1999;8(5):395-407.

[23] McCord G, Gilchrist VJ, Grossman SD, King BD, McCormick KF, Oprandi AM, et al. Discussing spirituality with patients: a rational and ethical approach. Annals of family medicine. 2004;2(4):356-61.

[24] Ehman JW, Ott BB, Short TH, Ciampa RC, Hansen-Flaschen J. Do patients want physicians to inquire about their spiritual or religious beliefs if they become gravely ill? Archives of Internal Medicine. 1999;159(15):1803-6.

[25] Luckhaupt SE, Yi MS, Mueller CV, Mrus JM, Peterman AH, Puchalski CM, et al. Beliefs of primary care residents regarding spirituality and religion in clinical encounters with patients: a study at a Midwestern US teaching institution. Academic Medicine. 2005;80(6):560-70.

[26] Monroe MH, Bynum D, Susi B, Phifer N, Schultz L, Franco M, et al. Primary care physician preferences regarding spiritual behavior in medical practice. Archives of Internal Medicine. 2003;163(22):2751-6.

[27] Ellis MR, Vinson DC, Ewigman B. Addressing spiritual concerns of patients: family physicians' attitudes and practices. The Journal of family practice. 1999;48(2):105-9.

[28] Schuster MA, Stein BD, Jaycox LH, Collins RL, Marshall GN, Elliott MN, et al. A national survey of stress reactions after the September 11, 2001, terrorist attacks. New England Journal of Medicine. 2001;345(20):1507-12.

[29] Ellis MR, Campbell JD, Detwiler-Breidenbach A, Hubbard DK. What do family physicians think about spirituality in clinical practice? Journal of Family Practice. 2002;51(3):249-58.

[30] Puchalski C, Romer A. Taking a spiritual history allows clinicians to understand patients more fully. Journal of Palliative Medicine. 2000;3(1):129-37.

[31] Anandarajah G, Hight E. Spirituality and medical practice: using the HOPE questions as a practical tool for spiritual assessment. American Family Physician. 2001;63(1):81-92.

[32] Koenig H. An 83-year-old woman with chronic illness and strong religious beliefs. Jama. 2002;288(4):487.

[33] Hodge D. A template for spiritual assessment: A review of the JCAHO requirements and guidelines for implementation. Social Work. 2006;51(4):317-26.

[34] Maugans T. The spiritual history. Archives of Family Medicine. 1996;5(1):11.

[35] Larocca-Pitts M. FACT: Taking a Spiritual History in a Clinical Setting. Journal of Health Care Chaplaincy. 2008;15(1):1-12.

[36] Lo B, Quill T, Tulsky J. Discussing palliative care with patients. Annals of Internal Medicine. 1999;130(9):744.

[37] Pargament KI, Murray-Swank NA, Magyar GM, Ano GG. Spiritual Struggle: A Phenomenon of Interest to Psychology and Religion. In: Delaney WMH, editor. Judeo-Christian perspectives on psychology: Human nature, motivation, and change. Washington DC: APA Press; 2005.

[38] Pargament KI, Koenig HG, Tarakeshwar N, Hahn J. Religious struggle as a predictor of mortality among medically ill elderly patients: a 2-year longitudinal study. Archives of Internal Medicine. 2001;161(15):1881-5.

[39] McConnell KM, Pargament KI, Ellison CG, Flannelly KJ. Examining the links between spiritual struggles and symptoms of psychopathology in a national sample. Journal of clinical psychology. 2006;62(12):1469-84.

[40] Ai AL, Seymour EM, Tice TN, Kronfol Z, Bolling SF. Spiritual struggle related to plasma interleukin-6 prior to cardiac surgery. Psychology of Religion and Spirituality. 2009;1(2):112-28.

[41] Daaleman TP. Religion, spirituality, and the practice of medicine. The Journal of the American Board of Family Medicine. 2004;17(5):370-6.

[42] Mueller PS, Plevak DJ, Rummans TA. Religious involvement, spirituality, and medicine: implications for clinical practice. Mayo Clinic Proceedings. 2001;76:1225-35.

[43] Daaleman TP, VandeCreek L. Placing religion and spirituality in end-of-life care. JAMA: the journal of the American Medical Association. 2000;284(19):2514-7.

[44] Azambuja LEOd, Garrafa V. Testemunhas de jeová ante o uso de hemocomponentes e hemoderivados. Revista da Associação Médica Brasileira. 2010;56:705-9.

[45] Curlin FA, Hall DE. Strangers or Friends?: A Proposal for a New Spirituality-in-Medicine Ethic. Journal of general internal medicine. 2005;20(4):370-4.

[46] Bell IR, Caspi O, Schwartz GER, Grant KL, Gaudet TW, Rychener D, et al. Integrative medicine and systemic outcomes research: issues in the emergence of a new model for primary health care. Archives of Internal Medicine. 2002;162(2):133-40.

[47] 58 th World Health Assembly.WHO Panel Report: Spirituality, Religion and Social Health. 2005; Available from: http://www.rcrescendo.org/11.Siritualitetpastorale/GINEBRA/SPIRITUALITY.pdf.

[48] McNutt LA, Waltermaurer E, McCauley J, Campbell J, Ford D. Rationale for and development of the computerized intimate partner violence screen for primary care. Family Violence Prevention and Health Practice. 2005;3:1-13.

[49] Lucchetti G, Granero A. Spirituality and Health's Most Productive Researchers: The Role of Primary Care Physicians. Family medicine. 2010;42(9):656-7.

[50] Larimore WL. Providing basic spiritual care for patients: should it be the exclusive domain of pastoral professionals? American family physician. 2001;63(1):36-8.

5

Telehealth: General Aspects in Primary Care

Alaneir de Fátima dos Santos, Humberto José Alves,
Cláudio de Souza, Simone Ferreira dos Santos,
Rosália Morais Torres and Maria do Carmo Barros de Melo
Telehealth Center, School of Medicine, Federal University of Minas Gerais
Brasil

1. Introduction

The World Health Organization (WHO, 2007) is confident that the major expectations regarding public health will be met in the 21st century as a result of improved access to resources – both qualitatively and quantitatively, which will then be available to most of the world population. Building on the assumption that the technological development has yielded significant contributions to the health field, particularly by facilitating knowledge sharing and promoting care education and training either in remote and isolated areas, WHO encourages its members to adopt telehealth as a politic and strategic tool to plan and implement health actions worldwide.

Telehealth programs have reached a wide range of distinct populations through a number of forms of Information and Communication Technology (ICT) aiming at health care professionals' qualification and continuing education, as well as accessibility, cost-efficiency and quality in health care services provided in both developed and developing countries.

In 2005 the World Health Organization created the Global Observatory for eHealth aiming at both revising the use of ICT in the health care field and assessing the benefits it provides in terms of health care and quality health assistance. In 2009, a WHO report showed progress after a few years investing in telehealth-based activities (Goe, 2010).

A number of successful experiences have been reported not only by WHO, but also in the literature within the health care domain, irrespective of their focus on assistance, therapy, education or diagnosis. Given this background of health "globalization", professionals involved with communication and information within the health care domain are now called upon to play an important role in promoting well-being, health care and happiness among patients and their relatives. Besides, their services particularly involve respecting ethical, moral and judicial standards, and assuring information privacy and confidentiality.

The WHO has adopted the following broad description for the term of telemedicine:

"The delivery of health care services, where distance is a critical factor, by all health care professionals using information and communication technologies for the exchange of valid information for

diagnosis, treatment and prevention of diseases and injuries, research and evaluation, and for continuing education of health care providers, all in the interest of advancing the health of individuals and the communities".

Four elements are germane to telemedicine:

1. Its purpose is to provide clinical support;
2. It is intended to overcome geographical barriers, connecting users who are not in the same physical location;
3. It involves the use of various types of ICT;
4. Its goal is to improve health outcomes. (Goe, 2010)

The term "telehealth" have been currently applied in the literature in reference to any health care services, ranging from prevention to treatment and rehabilitation. The term has been used in the broad sense, and given it accommodates several activities across the health care field it has been associated with the idea of interdisciplinarity.

On the other hand, the term eHealth or e-Health has been used since the year 2000, especially in publications and institutional documents. That is the case, for instance, of the major international organizations, such as WHO, the European Union (UE), the International Telecommunication Union (ITU), and the European Space Agency. Different definitions of the term eHealth suggest different functions, institutional partnerships, contexts and theoretical and expected goals.

Eysenbach (2001) for instance, defines it as:

"e-health is an emerging field of medical informatics, referring to the organization and delivery of health services and information using the Internet and related technologies. In a broader sense, the term characterizes not only a technical development, but also a new way of working, an attitude, and a commitment for networked, global thinking, to improve health care locally, regionally, and worldwide by using information and communication technology."

eHealth have been used in a number of ways, changing according to the need and the tools involved. The current processes are: teleconsultation, telediagnosis, second-opinion medical advice, telesurgery, telemonitoring (telesurveillance), tele-education (continuing education), clinical simulation, electronic medical report, databank compilation and analysis, virtual image libraries, and so on.

The use of computation and telecommunication has been increasingly expanding in the public health area, involving research activities and following technology developments within both developed and developing countries.

m-Health programs have been designed for mobile electronic devices (MED), such as personal digital assistants (PADs) and mobile phones, aiming at supporting clinical decision-making, ensuring reliable data collection and promoting changes in patients' behaviors that impact on health care promotion and management of chronic diseases in the community (Free *et al.*, 2010).

Mobile telecommunication has the advantage of covering areas that are not covered by regular Internet carriers, besides being useful for travelers, who have been already reported to send tomography images and electrocardiograms (Hernett, 2006).

The easier access to Internet has contributed to such practices involving texts, images and sounds that can be sent quite quickly. A number of devices are available, such as mobile phones, PDAs, Smartphones, e-Books, portable or ultraportable computers.

The literature reports on several m-health applications, including, but not limited to: short message service (SMS) to support the control of chronic diseases, such as diabetes, hypertension, asthma, eating disorders, and HIV treatment; SMS and PAD messages to support the control of tobaccoism, weight loss, and alcoholism. The latter have been used to collect data for research, to promote health care and to support medical education and clinical practices (Free *et al.*, 2010).

The current distance education relies on the use of multimedia, including printed materials, CDs, DVDs, televisions, web-connected computers, didactic videos and even online simulators. Teaching-learning technology has increasingly relied upon the online transmission of data, voice and image via satellite or optical fiber, and it has particularly focused on the interaction between students and the distance education centers, this interaction being mediated either by artificial intelligence or by the online communication between students, teachers and tutors (Guaranys & Castro, 1979).

Currently, a number of countries, such as Mexico, Tanzania, Nigeria, Angola and Mozambique, have adopted distance education strategies in a large scale to train their teachers and other professionals, including those in the fields of health care, agriculture, and social security, in both public and health organizations. Particularly in Brazil, a great number of technicians and financial resources have been allocated to distance education, both in public organizations and in private companies, in the last few decades. The results have pointed to several positive outcomes, but also to some difficulties and shortcomings. Most of them are related to discontinued projects, lack of coherence and continuity in public administration, and political and cultural difficulties to apply more solid criteria and scientific methodologies to assess programs and projects (Nunes, 1992).

Telemonitoring of patients with chronic diseases is also an expanding activity worldwide. It enables professionals to better control their patients and to provide both patients and their relatives with disease-specific pieces of information. The expected result is reduced morbi-mortality and hospital admissions, and the ultimate goal is to place patients under the care of primary care teams.

Health care based on Family and Community Medicine can qualitatively improve with electronic medical management, support systems for clinical decision-making and adequate information flow from family and community doctors to other professionals in the health care systems, and vice-versa. The new technologies urge the physician to face new ethical issues regarding safety and reliability, privacy and exposure, as well as globalization of knowledge and clinical practices (Kvist & Kidd, 2010).

As globalization moves on uninterruptedly, knowledge sharing increases with the support of ICT tools. If authorities, researchers and the population itself gather efforts, telehealth may help overcome physical, economic and social barriers and thus promote equitable assistance at all levels of health care (Melo & Silva, 2008).

To be sure, telehealth improves the effectiveness of public health and primary care interventions, as it contributes to train health care professionals and improves the delivery of health services.

The WHO (2008) identifies significant changes in the health context worldwide: 1) The remarkable health advances have been meaningfully unequal; 2) the nature of health problems have been changing on a hardly predictable and unexpected pace as a result of new social, demographic and epidemiological patterns emerged with globalization, urbanization, and population ageing processes; and 3) the new health systems are also responsive to the pace of changes in the current globalization process.

Besides the existence of a number of non-regulated commercial health care services, the thin limits between the roles and accountabilities of public and private agents are not clear, and the negotiation of licenses and rights serve political interests. Exclusively commercial, non-regulated health services are usually inefficient and costing, exacerbates inequality and provide poor quality (sometimes, dangerous) health care. Health care merchandization affects reliability of health care services and the population's trust in the authorities' capacity to protect society.

Three alarming tendencies have been observed among health services worldwide: 1) Cure-oriented health systems focusing on specialized health care; 2) fragmented health services focusing on some diseases and short-term results; and 3) health systems based on non-intervention or laissez-faire policies, which leaves room for commercial health care (Eysenbach, 2001).

The World Health Organization also stresses that despite increased resources over the last ten years, several countries suffer from lack of resources in the health sector. As a result, such countries miss the opportunity to promote structural changes and build more efficient and equitable systems. Health policies have been unresponsive and from time to time establish one short-term priority or another, which shows their increasingly fragmented nature and lack of long-term perspective.

In the international context, health systems focusing on primary care have been proved to reduce costs and improve morbi-mortality irrespective of social classes. Such focus, aligned with increasing investments on health care above Gross Domestic Product (GDP) and population growth, has promoted a twofold agenda converging to primary health.

On the one hand, WHO restates values embedded in the Declaration of Alma-Ata, stressing that the protection and promotion of the health of all the people of the world demands health systems sensitive to both the challenges of an ever-changing world and the expectation of better results. This implies a need of substantial restructure and reform of the current health systems, which constitutes the grounds of the primary care renewal agenda (WHO, 2008). According to WHO, such a renewal meets the population's needs of expectations towards more socially relevant services that are not only more sensitive to the world's change, but also produce better results.

On the other hand, the liberal model has been moving the agenda to include changes in more restrict functional dimensions, especially with regards to costs: a) Selective packages focusing on service offer under the primary health care principals as prescribed by the World Bank for poor or developing countries; and b) managed care, which presupposes first contact services before patients are referred to specialists or more complex procedures as well as large use of information technologies to control costs.

Such model gained significance in the 1990s, when it influenced the structure of several health systems. New initiatives, however, were implemented later on, especially in Europe. Such changes have yielded significant improvements on primary care quality and efficiency (Giovanella & Mendoça, 2008). Some of them have led to more power and control of primary care providers over providers of other levels of care (such as coordinator and buyer) and others have enlarged the range of functions and serviced supplied and offered at the primary level, thus expanded the providers' role to include new curative actions, mental health community services, home care and palliative care, besides the implementation of information and communication systems, as well as continuing education.

Primary care implementation has had a deep, dynamic impact on the tendency in the health systems, as it has introduced new resources allocation modalities, changed education, the workplace and service organization, exerted pressure on the decentralization process, and enhanced popular participation (Kinfu et al., 2005).

As observed in very successful experiences in some countries, health care implementation not only is important as a door for further referral, but also has the potential to serve as a key element for the strategic sustainability of health systems as it helps coordinate secondary and tertiary healthcare.

It is in this context of health systems focusing on primary care that the telehealth resources must be understood. Primary care is thus assumed as the level of care that: 1) is the gateway for the population's needs and problems and provides care to people over time; 2) provides care for any health conditions, apart from those that are very uncommon or rare; and 3) coordinates or integrates health care provided somewhere else or by third parties.

Planning telehealth to provide both permanent education and support to professional teams of primary care-oriented programs does reinforce the key role of primary care in the health systems.

Some projects implemented in such level of care, linking primary health care units with high education units in the areas of nursing, dentistry and medicine enable, primary care professionals to discuss clinical cases with professors and also to participate in videoconferences whereby they can discuss the most relevant care problems at this level of care.

The introduction of telehealth grants primary care professionals with the access to specialists to discuss clinical case in order to either improve the services they provide to a given patient or to opt for further referral to a specialist. In other words, the professionals have their capacity expanded and become more qualified for the service they provide.

Projects involving distance-learning webconferences are innovative in content and technology, but most importantly they offer a special learning dynamics in which the feeling of belonging to a virtual community does play an important role for the learners. Learning competences therefore builds on the introduction of group-oriented efficient and innovative practices. It is the group that plays the role of interlocutor in the webconferences, it is the group that builds its own identify in the community of practice and it is the group that becomes strong through mechanisms of evaluation and acceptance of new care practices.

The feeling of belonging to a virtual community where peer can share experiences and ways of work set the context for the skills to be learnt by the health teams, which is important in a process of changing attitudes and accountabilities regarding health care.

The fact that webconferences are based on actual care problems faced by health professionals implies an actual process of experience sharing, not only between professors and professionals, but also among the professionals themselves.

Differently from managed care, which focuses on real-time work to put new health practices in place (Mehry, 2011), telehealth projects open up a range of new possibilities to support clinical decision making both at the primary level of care and across the different levels. The result is a more qualified primary level of care along with increased control of referral to the next level, as health care teams have already carried out a number of preliminary analyses and also taken the necessary measures for which they are accountable.

The logic is turned upside down: It is the secondary and tertiary levels of care that help to keep patients at the primary level, and the decentralized referral mechanism ensures that most of the work is done at the primary level. The introduction of telehealth resources:

1.   Optimizes the primary level role in coordinating how health care is provided to patients. As the discussion of actual and specific clinical cases inform primary care professionals they have the necessary knowledge to only make referral of patients that do need health care at other levels. This introduces a new way to provide health services: professional share their diagnoses and assessments before making referral of patients to other levels of care, which is a key procedure to develop more effective and integrated health care networks;
2.   Enhances the primary level of care, as it enlarges the scope of this level: Primary care professionals are empowered to follow up patients even in more complex cases, as they share knowledge and information with specialists instead of simply referring patients to them;
3.   Enables follow up under different circumstances: even when patients are referred, the primary care professionals have full understanding of their situation and take the first measures to treat a given patient. Knowledge sharing is a key step to bring the different levels of care together;
4.   provides continuing education, so primary care professionals can learn from actual cases and be empowered to provide more complex health care treatments with the help of professionals working at the secondary and tertiary levels.

In practice, introducing telehealth resources contribute to place primary health care as the foundation that supports and determines the activities at all levels of care within the health systems. It is healthcare itself the foundation that organizes and rationalizes all the resources (both basic and specialized) oriented to promote, maintain and improve health (Starfield, 2002).

In the broad context of primary care renewal to cope with the new challenges of an ever-changing world, the introduction of telehealth resources serves to develop a more rational process of both cutting and allocating costs without either affecting quality or controlling physicians' performance. On the contrary, knowledge sharing is a key tool to introduce new elements in health care services that are more likely to generate successful results and avoid unnecessary costs.

It does interfere in the health and medical system as whole, but it is highly expected to generate positive impacts on how health care services are delivered, as it draws on primary care and people networking.

By identifying the necessary primary care renewals, reforms are supposed, as WHO stresses, to aim at universal health coverage that ensure equality, social justice, end of social exclusion, and social protection to health. Such renewals should embrace three perspectives: 1) Coverage expansion, i.e. to expand the parcel of the population that enjoys social protection to health; 2) Coverage enhancement, i.e. to expand the range of health services in order to provide for the population's needs efficiently and meet demands and expectations, but also taking into account the resources the society is both willing and capable to afford; 3) Coverage level, i.e. to eliminate direct payment for the services.

Taking such perspectives into account, telehealth resources can contribute to at least two of them, as telehealth is a potential tool to expand and enhance coverage, especially in those areas for which no specialists are available. Furthermore, the introduction of telehealth resources in patient's homes especially to monitor such chronic pathologies as hypertension and diabetes has generated new care modalities to face the impact of demographic transition, which makes the co-morbidity process more complex.

Therefore, in the light of challenges in the way to provide universal and equitable coverage as preconized by WHO, telehealth services is expected to contribute as follows: 1) To gradually create primary care networks to remedy the lack of services available; 2) To overcome the isolation of scattered populations; 3) To address inequality issues related to health; and 4) To open avenues for civil societies' participation and empowerment.

The use of telehealth resources can also contribute in the process of health reforms aiming at shifting from the conventional health system to a primary care-oriented health system that is more socially pertinent and responsive to current changes in the world. Several international experiences have been successful in allying information technology with distance health services via telehealth as the patients' first contact with the health systems.

Telehealth can also help and integrate actions aiming at policy reforms targeting a series of policies to face challenges posed by urbanization, climatic change, epidemiological profiles and social stratification. In other words, telehealth resources can be a key tool for the society, especially when it integrates several healthcare dimensions within the health systems.

2. Key benefits of the use of telehealth

Telehealth appears as an important tool for the actions recommended for health promotion to be implemented (Norris, 2002; Wooton et al., 2005; Stroetmann, 2010). Nonetheless, there is a lack of robust data on the clinical effectiveness, the risks of the implementation of the telehealth technologies and their cost-effectiveness (Ekeland et al., 2010; Black, 2011).

The following main actions and products that can be achieved to improve primary health care (Table 1) are based mainly in preliminary pilot project results, opinions and prediction.

Actions	Benefits for primary care
Telemonitoring of chronic illnesses	Better disease control; Reduction of comorbidity and mortality; Improved quality of life; Reduction in hospital admissions and demand for emergency care services; Reduced absenteeism; Reduction of public expenditure on hospitalization and sequels.
Second opinion via teleconsultation	Health professionals retention in rural areas; Improved patient assistance; Better health care professional/patient ratio; Reduced patient traveling; Opportunity to share knowledge; Access to specialists improving clinical decision making; Reduction of waiting times for consultation with specialists.
Videoconferencing	In service training of professionals; Opportunity to share doubts and decisions.
eLearning	Training with less traveling; Social Interaction; Shared space of knowledge construction and development; Constructive and critical support through tutoring.

Table 1. Telehealth tools and potential products in primary health care

3. The Brazilian experience

The reorganization of the health system in Brazil, including the focus on primary health care, has been recent. The implementation has relied upon professionals who have traditionally had a conventional educational background, with courses structured according to a highly specialized, curative, individual and hospital centered approach. The challenge of incorporating telehealth resources in the Brazilian public system (SUS – *Sistema Único de Saúde* in Portuguese) is linked to the objective of strengthening the public model already established. It also had the intention of reinforcing the role of primary health care in a context where professionals are still not adequately trained, both from the point of view of dealing with clinical issues at this level of attention and of promoting health.

The National Telehealth Program currently consists of 1,011 telehealth centers connected to 10 universities and spread over 789 municipalities, benefiting some 2,796 health family teams. One of the dimensions of this project is based on the webconferences. In a State of Minas Gerais webconferences addressing family health teams within member municipalities take place every 15 days and involve classes and talks given by professionals in the areas of medicine, nursing and dentistry. A multicast network transmits the talks simultaneously to multiple Primary Health Care Units in the municipalities. A multipoint videoconference software package enables telecommunication resources comprising images, data and voice as well as shared electronic medical records. The virtual learning environment reproduces a classroom simultaneously offering audio, video, data and graphic resources in a group-friendly learning-oriented environment.

The Telehealth Center of Medicine School at Federal University of Minas Gerais (NUTEL) in partnership with the programs BHtelehealth and the Brazilian National Telehealth Program has developed activities involving teleconsultation, teleassistance, videoconference and distance education, and it is currently designing projects to telemonitor diabetic and hypertensive patients and follow up asthmatic patients. The following education centers participate in NUTEL activities: School of Medicine, School of Dentistry, School of Nursing, and Laboratory of Scientific Computation of the Federal University of Minas Gerais (UFMG – *Universidade Federal de Minas Gerais* in Portuguese)

NUTEL has its own team to produce instructional materials, including videos, animations, 2D and 3D modeling, and this team has contributed to design distance courses and instructional materials to be published by the Brazilian Ministry of Health and several Municipality Health Departments. The material has supported training programs focusing on health care projects and also educational programs focusing the community, particularly aiming at the control and prevention of epidemics and infectious diseases, such as H1N1 and Dengue. Part of the materials is also distributed among private corporations. The distance education courses offered by NUTEL include: Urgency and Emergency, Electrocardiogram Interpretation, Arterial Hypertension, Dengue, Chagas' Disease, Diabetes, Arterial Hypertension during Pregnancy, Traumas. NUTEL is also developing courses on Childhood Asthma and Telehealth for Policy Makers of Latin American countries involved in an Inter-American Development Bank (IDB)-funded project, "Regional Public Policies on Telehealth in Latin America and the Caribbean ".

Distance education is an important educational strategy that responds to the needs of a large number of professionals that are not able or willing to move from one place to another. It is more effective than several other teaching modalities that exclusively demand student's physical presence, irrespective of the number of students attending the courses. It meets current demands of universal education both efficiently and qualitatively, representing an adequate source of knowledge update in a world in ongoing change. It is an efficient solution to a number of barriers that primary health care professionals may face when it comes to pursuing continuing education, including limited budgets, schedules, on-the-job learning opportunities, access to information and offer of services by public institutions (Mathauer & Imhoff, 2006). Furthermore, continuing education is crucial for physicians living and working in remote areas, as it increases self-confidence and reduces professional isolation, which are key elements to attach them to these unprivileged areas.

NUTEL currently offers online and offline teleconsultation systems with a team of professionals on duty providing services on internal medicine, pediatrics, gynecology, obstetrics, dermatology, dentistry, nursing, physiotherapy, pharmacy, nutrition and clinical pathology, besides access to over 46 medical specialists. Professionals working in family health teams are allowed to access the system, whereby they can describe a particular clinical case on the basis of either a real situation or a context-free question. They can also attach images and other files that assumedly help understand the case (diagnosis, propaedeutic, and therapy). The teleconsultants analyze every request and reply them according to a system-generated priority list.

Every piece of information is protected through a number of methods, including cryptography, message integrity, user authentication, and safe backup policy. Every user has a nontransferable personal login and password that expires within a given limit of time.

Videoconferences and webconferences have taken place both domestically and internationally, focusing on primary health care as promoted by UFMG School of Nursing, School of Dentistry and School of Medicine. Some of them have been provided in partnership with BHTelehealth Program and the National Telehealth Program.

In 2003, the city of Belo Horizonte, known for its innovation and success in the organization of the Brazilian National Health System (SUS), prepared a project to incorporate ICT. The process (BHTelehealth project) reflected the objective of providing the assistance model, centered on primary health care, the necessary tools for strengthening the quality of attention. In addition, it sought to structure the educational training of the professionals by using innovative distance learning resources such as interactive environments, organic modeling in 3D, animations and videos. It sought to create a process of permanent education for its professionals and staff that would include the use of interactive resources, 3D modeling and animations in distance learning courses, teleconsultations and videoconferences.

The National Telehealth Program assigned an expert group to analyze interactivity solutions available in the market and then point out the pros and cons of each software package. Their report provided enough information for each center to opt for software package that would be most suitable for their needs. The Telehealth Center at the UFMG School of Medicine adopts the copyright packages Sametime® and Adobe Connect®.

One of the challenges posed by the webconferences is the design of a curriculum that do meet the actual health demand detected by the health family teams. To face this challenge, NUTEL has defined the curriculum topics during the webconferences that promotes with the municipalities in the State of Minas Gerais in the beginning of every semester. Table 2 shows the number of participants attending the webconferences in the State of Minas Gerais from 2008 through 2010, as provided by the very webconference software package. This is a way to ensure that the topics approached in the webconferences address the problems identified by the technical coordinators and the health professionals themselves. Among the most frequent topics are complex problems identified in the delivery of primary care services or in unexpected epidemiologic situations.

Area/Year	2008	2009	2010
Medicine	590	513	594
Nursing	1149	676	926
Dentistry	1217	605	904
Total	2956	1794	2424

Source: Nutel/UFMG.

Table 2. Webconference participants of the National Telehealth Program, 2008 - 2010.

To be sure, the major objective of a webconference on primary health care is to ensure professionals' learning on the basis of the very problems they identify in the course of their professional activities.

Distance education is still an incipient activity in Brazil, but some initiatives have opened doors to turn it into a large-scale public policy in the country. The main ongoing initiatives aim at improving any given dimension of the primary health care. They are carried out in the framework of the National Telehealth Program and the Open University/Brazilian Health System (UNA/SUS in Portuguese), which shows the Ministry of Health's concern with framing primary care as the organization and coordination dimension of the health care services delivered to the population. The recent institutional status given to UNA/SUS in late 2010 is a landmark that will boost the design and implementation of health-oriented distance learning courses, as UNA/SUS is now assigned to plan and coordinate the leading initiatives in the area. On the other hand, the initiatives implemented by the National Telehealth Program has already helped a number of Brazilian states experience the potential of new teaching technologies, as particularly observed in regard to the webconferences and the courses, the latter also aggregating market power given the use of simulators, organic modeling and animations. This process focusing on training professors from the major public universities and health professionals in Brazil has helped introduce the potentials of this technology in the health field.

The webconferences and teleconsultations have been important activities to both training family health teams and to improve the health care services delivered to the population without the health professionals' need to commute in order to receive formal education.

The referral of patients from primary health care professionals to specialists is considerably difficult in the national health systems, as they have no time slots in their schedules. Patients' commuting is also difficult, because of intense traffic flow in the Brazilian roads, inadequate road maintenance, high costs and large distances within the Brazilian territory. Besides the delivery of better health care services, teleconsultations are a key tool to spread knowledge among professionals and reduce isolation feelings among those living and working in remote and rural areas. Patients have reported satisfaction when they get to know specialist and professors are discussing their cases, and this reinforces their empathy and ties with the family health teams.

The telemonitoring of hypertensive and diabetic patients is an incipient project within the National Telehealth Program. The idea is to use the existing telehealth structure to monitor and follow up glucose and arterial pressure in patients in serious condition. This patients will be monitored by their health family teams and a specialist particularly gathered for this purpose at UFMG School of Medicine and School of Nursing. This will eventually result in teleconsultations scheduled in advance, continuous networking among members of the health family teams, and implementation of learning courses based on reliable simulators and experimented levels of difficulty. Simultaneously, training courses, simulators and videoconferences will provide an in-depth approach to the process preconized by the Brazilian Ministry of Health for the monitoring of these pathologies by the heath family teams. All the municipalities will participate in this training process, and the 50 primary health units selected for the monitoring activities will also have their activities implemented in order to provide such follow up accordingly. By the end of two years, it is expected to have a very well structured process to monitor hypertensive and diabetic patients within the primary care framework. This will be based on the telehealth strategy, which will possibly go through an in-depth assessment.

4. Future of telehealth in primary care

Currently primary care is internationally considered the basis for a new model of user-citizen centered health care systems. In European countries, primary care refers generally to outpatient services first with an integrated system of universal access. At a conference in Alma-Ata, primary care was seen as essential health care based on practical, scientifically sound and socially acceptable methods and technology, the first component of an ongoing process of health care, access to which should be fully guaranteed for the entire population (Giovanella & Mendonça, 2008).

The Bangkok Charter for Health Promotion in a Globalized World (2005), identifies actions, commitments and pledges required to address the determinants of health in a globalized world through health promotion. Emphasizes that globalization opens up new opportunities for cooperation to improve health and reduce transnational health risks. These new opportunities include:

- optimization of information and communication technology;
- improvement of governance processes and sharing of experiences.

The future of information and communication technology in primary care is beneficial and should be present in the medical and other health professionals, prescription, guidelines and telemonitoring. The electronic health record (HER) and teleconsultation are already a reality. Also the support for the diagnosis and therapeutic decision making with the help of mobile phones, through the consultation of electronic documents, allowing them access to some protocols and scores, doses and drug prescriptions. The telemonitoring is possible with the use of mobile equipment (mHealth) or through home computers with the possibility of access to tests and verification of the adherence to treatment (Speedie et al., 2008; Stroetmann, 2010).

5. Conclusion

Nowadays health services management can use telehealth resources making possible the integration of services and opening up new possibilities for training professionals in remote areas. As a result health professionals feel their work is more valued, increasing the opportunities for them to remain in the remote regions away from large urban centers. Also, services provided to the population have a significant improvement in quality, since telehealth technology allows health professionals to have an increased online and offline interaction with other centers.

The use of telehealth resources in primary care is in expansion, with varied application levels that include activities ranging from tele-education to teleconsultation, second opinion telemonitoring and telecare. Since the education process happens at the health unit, it implies in efforts optimization and resources rationalization, once professionals do not have to move from his/her workplace.

Considering the assistance aspects for municipalities, the possibility of health professionals discussing clinical cases with specialists increases the effectiveness and adds quality to the primary care. Objective and subjective evaluations of the benefits that come with this data is a complex process, which is under development in the program. Concerning the second opinion, its usage contributes to structure the assistance models linked with different complexity levels. The use of telehealth resources on these remote areas introduces a change in the working process.

6. References

Black A.D., Car J., Pagliari C., Anandan C., Cresswell K., Bokun T., McKinstry B., Procter R., Majeed A. & Sheikh A. 2011. The impact of ehealth on the quality and safety of health care: a systematic overview. PLoS Medicine, Vo.8, No.1:e1000387. Retrieved from http://www.plosmedicine.org/article/info%3Adoi%2F10.1371%2Fjournal.pmed.1 000387

Ekeland A.G., Bowes A. & Flottrop S. 2010. *International Journal on Medical Informatics* Effectiviness of telemedicine: a systematic review of reviews, Vo.79, pp.736-771, ISSN 1386-5056.

Eysenbach G. 2001;What is e-health? *Journal of Medical Internet Research*, Vo. 3, No.2:e20. Retrieved from http://www.jmir.org/2001/2/e20/

Free C., Phillips G., Felix L., Galli L., Patel V. & Edwards P. 2010. BMC Research Notes, Vo. 3:250. Access Feb. 26. Available from: http://www.ncbi.nlm.nih.gov/pmc/articles/PMC2976743/pdf/1756-0500-3-250.pdf

Giovanella L.& Mendonça M.H.M. 2008. Atenção primária em saúde. In: *Políticas e sistemas de saúde no Brasil*. Giovanella L., Escorel S., Lobato L.V.C., Noronha J.C., Carvalho A.I. pp.575-625, Editora Vera Cruz, ISBN 978-85-7541-157-5, Rio de Janeiro.

Guaranys L.R. & Castro C.M. 1979. O ensino por correspondência: uma estratégia de desenvolvimento educacional no Brasil. *IPEA*, ISSN 167-6079.

Hernett B. Telemedicine systems and telecommunications. 2006. In: *Introduction to Telemedicine*. Wootton R., Craig J. & Patterson V. pp. 15-34. Royal of Medicine Press Ltd., ISBN 1853156779, London.

Kinfu Y., Dal Poz M.R., Mercer H. & Evans D.B. 2009. The health worker shortage in Africa: are enough physicians and nurses being trained? *Bulletin of World Health Organization*,Vo. 87, pp. 225–230. ISSN 0042-9686.

Kvist M. & Kidd M. 2010. O papel das novas tecnologias da informação e comunicação na atenção primária. In: *Atenção Primária conduzindo as redes de atenção à saúde – Reforma organizacional na atenção primária européia*. Saltman R.B., Rico A., Boerma W.G.W. pp. 317-338, Open university press. ISBN 13978033521365 8, England.

Mathauer I. & Imhoff I. 2006. Health worker motivation in Africa: the role of non-financial incentives and human resource management tools. *Human Resource for Health*, Vo. 4, pp. 24–41, ISSN 14784491.

Melo M.C.B. & Silva E.M.S. 2006. Aspectos conceituais em telessaúde. In: *Telessaúde*, Santos A.F., Souza C., Alves H.J., Santos S.F, pp. 17-31, Ed. UFMG, Belo Horizonte, ISBN 8570415826.

Merhy E.E. 2001. E daí surge o PSF como uma continuidade e um aperfeiçoamento do PACS. *Interface Comunicação, saúde e educação*, Vo.9, pp.147-149, ISSN 1414-3283.

Nunes I.B. 1992. Educação à Distância e o Mundo do Trabalho. *Tecnologia Educacional.* Vol.21, No. 107, jul/ago, pp. 73-74, ISSN 0102-5503.

Norris A.C. 2002. *Essentials of telemedicine and telecare.* John Wiley & Sons Ltda, ISBN 0470851813, England.

Speedie S.M., Ferguson S., Sanders J. & Doarn C.R. 2008. Telehealth: the promise of the new care delivery models. *Telemedicine and e-Health,* Vo.14, No.9, pp.964-967, ISSN 15305627.

Starfield B. 2002. *Atenção primária: equilíbrio entre necessidade de saúde, serviços e tecnologia.* Brasília: UNESCO/Ministério da Saúde. Retrieved from http://bvsms.saude.gov.br/bvs/publicacoes/atencao_primaria_p1.pdf

Stroetmann K.A., Kubitschke L., Robinson S., Stroetmann V., Cullen K. & McDaid D. 2010, How can telehealth help in the provision of integrated care? *World Health Organization,* Copenhagen. Retrieved from http://www.euro.who.int/__data/assets/pdf_file/0011/120998/E94265.pdf

Wootton R., Craig J. & Paterson V. 2006. *Introduction to telemedicine.* 2nd ed. Royal Society of Medicine Press Ltd, ISBN 1853156779. London, UK.

World Health Organization. The Bangkok Charter for Health Promotion in a Globalized World, Bangkok, Thailand, 2005. (http://www.who.int/healthpromotion/conferences/6gchp/hpr_050829_%20BCHP.pdf -accessed 9 november 2011).

World Health Organization. Department of essential health technologies. Information technology in support of health care. Genebra, [s.d.]. Access Sept. 07 2007. Available from: < www.who.int/entity/eht/en/InformationTech.pdf >

World Health Organization. The World Health Report 2008 - primary Health Care. Access Nov. 11 2011. Available from: http://www.who.int/whr/2008/en/index.html

World Health Organization. Global Observatory for eHealth Series, 2. Telemedicine: opportunities and developments in Member States: report on the second global survey on eHealth, 2010. p.96.

6

Telemedicine in Primary Care

Jumana Antoun
American University of Beirut
Lebanon

1. Introduction

I receive a call from a parent telling me that his 4 year old has developed a rash. Despite all the questions about its shape and consistency, I was not confident to reassure the parent. Suddenly, he sends me a photo of the rash on my blackberry. Another parent audio recorded his child's cough that was bothering them all night. On daily basis, I see patients who present to the office for checkup from close adjacent countries. They are in a hurry and leave before the results of the tests are out, or they might do the tests when they go back to their own country. So I use email correspondence to comment on the results or receive the results. I have a depressed patient who still corresponds with me about her medical condition as she had to leave the country to continue her education. Every now and then, I am challenged with patients who want to discuss sensitive issues by emails like impotence or unusual obsessions. Definitely, you have encountered that meticulous patients who has jotted his blood pressure readings on an excel sheet, printed it and brought it to the clinic. The above scenarios are some aspects of telemedicine and they pose some questions to answer concerning the appropriateness of this way of communication; safety and assurance of confidentiality and privacy in communications, effectiveness, preference of patients.

Telemedicine is defined as the use of telecommunications technology to provide medical information and services to geographically distant population. As a result, telemedicine has tremendous applications in different domains of diagnosis, treatment, education and research and has been applied in dermatology, radiology, cardiology, surgery, etc. There exist two modes of operations: real-time and store-and-forward modes. In store-an-forward approach, the transmission is asynchronous and the recipient can access the data at a later time. It is used in transmission of photos of skin lesions, imaging studies, chronic disease measurements between health care providers or between the patient and health care provider for second opinion, specialist consultation or physician feedback. In real-time approach, both parties need to synchronize their time. It is used in videoconferencing, and telesurgery.

Most of the literature describe short termed pilot projects as there are number of barriers that hinder the fast adoption of such applications: 1) privacy and security; (2) reliability of information; (3) technological challenges such as bandwidth and interfacing; (4) the lack of technology and money in areas of utmost need of this technology; (5) cost; (6) lack of standards and interoperability. Moreover, there are certain challenges to teleconsultation mainly licensure, liability and legal issues; physicians who practice across different states or countries might be subject to different practices and thus exposed to lawsuits.

Despite the potential benefits of telemedicine in improving access, there is a need to establish the quality of the services and its impact on quality of care. A Cochrane review has shown that telemedicine applications are feasible yet enough evidence is still lacking concerning their effects on health outcomes or costs. (Currell et al., 2000) For example, in one study, transmitting x-ray radiographs to a remote orthopedic surgeon using the mobile phone MMS (multimedia messaging service) resulted in under or over diagnosing that would have led to mismanagement in 48% of the cases. (Chandhanayingyong et al., 2007) Definitely, there are some limitations to the accuracy of the physical exam using teleconsultation such as the lack of palpation and smell. (Boodley, 2006)

2. Telemedicine applications in primary care

2.1 Home monitoring for chronic disease management

Remote monitoring for disease management is one important application of telemedicine. Home telemonitoring systems have been implemented in many chronic diseases as asthma, chronic obstructive pulmonary disease (COPD), diabetes, hypertension and heart failure. A systematic review has shown that these systems are reliable and accurate with very few technical errors. (Pare et al., 2007) Telemonitoring projects had led to positive improvements in outcomes though the findings were not consistent across all projects and diseases. However, there are reported benefits of decrease in hemoglobin A1c, reduction in systolic and diastolic blood pressure, detection of early deterioration in COPD patients and decrease in hospital admissions. (Pare et al., 2007; Pare et al., 2010) In addition, use of home telemonitoring empowers the patients to actively get engaged in their care, and improving their general sense of well-being. (Pare et al., 2007)

Home telemonitoring requires monitoring hardware and software that will automatically record data from the patient such as weight, heart rate, blood glucose level, insulin use, etc. Some systems alert the provider and the patient to warning values; others are complemented with web-based information for self-support. Major barriers to remote monitoring include the cost of the equipment; need for personnel for installation and maintenance and system reliability; moreover the equipment should be simple and easily used by the patient and customized to an elderly population.

2.2 Web portals

More institutions and vendors are investing in providing Web based portal usage to their systems. This is driven by the total interconnectivity of the Internet on a global scale as well as the lower costs needed as data storage and maintenance is handled by the application service provider (ASP). Moreover, it will empower the patients as they get involved in health decisions. It has a promising future in improving communication between various parties such as physicians, hospitals and insurers thus providing a holistic care. A patient can log in to the portal and request prescription refills and referrals, have access to schedule an appointment, browse through the health library as well as send messages to their physician.

In a pilot study of implementation of Patient Gateway, physicians described their experience with using the web portal as positive in the administrative issues such as refill, referral and appointment requests. (Kittler et al., 2004) One important obstacle to the use of providers of such systems is their fear of increase in workload in the absence of reimbursement. (Kittler et al., 2004) In addition, lack of standards and interoperability among different sources of data pose a great challenge to the design of these portals.

2.3 Teleconsultation

Teleconsultation has been used more frequently between health care providers for specialist opinion or referral purposes. It requires more sophisticated equipment such as digital cameras, digital scopes, and videoconferencing facilities. Transmission of digital retinal images by primary care practitioner to ophthalmology specialist was as effective as personal evaluation for screening for diabetic retinopathy. This has tremendous benefits to diabetic patients or older patients who live in remote areas or can not visit multiple doctors for mobility limitations. There are few reported projects where teleconsultation occurred between patients and their providers. In a geriatric retiring community, most patients were able to use the computer system to communicate with their physician without assistance; the majority could accurately see and hear the health care provider. (Bratton & Cody, 2000)

3. Email communication

In this chapter, we will be discussing email communication between physician and patients based on contractual relationship that is the patient is known to the physician in contrast to emails communication in forum discussions.

3.1 Scope of use of email communication between patients and physicians

The practice of email communication between patients and providers lags tremendously behind the increase in the general email usage and willingness of patients to send email messages to their health care providers. (Sittig et al., 2001) Eighty five percent of 9000 email users surveyed in 2000 reported daily use of email; yet only 6% have even sent an email to their provider. (Sittig et al., 2001) Despite two thirds of university based clinic patients who access their emails almost daily at home or work, 90% have never used email communication with their physician. (Moyer et al., 2002a) Even in the past decade, the utilization of emails between patients and physician has modestly increased. A membership survey of the American College of physician - American Society of Internal medicine showed that less that 7% of internists (15,375 respondents) exchanged email communication with their patients on weekly or daily basis though two thirds had access to computers and used Internet from home for email uses. (Lacher et al., 2000) A study in 2006, 16.6% of 4203 Florida physicians used email from their office for communication with patients; 17.4% of those physicians (or 2.9% of the total number of physicians) used emails with patients on daily basis. (Brooks & Menachemi, 2006) A following survey representing the same population in 2008 revealed a slight increase in the percentage of physicians who use email (20%). (Menachemi et al., 2011)

3.2 Characteristics of physicians and patients who utilize email communication

In general, physicians who are early adopters of this email communication with patients are more than their counterpart to be enthusiastic about its usage and less bothered by time pressures. (Moyer et al., 2002a) Physicians who are more likely to use emails with their patients were younger, university based (Gaster et al., 2003), had training in family medicine or surgery and practiced in large groups of 50 or more. (Brooks & Menachemi, 2006) Older physicians (>60 years old) and physicians of Asian descent are unlikely to involve in email usage with their patients. (Brooks & Menachemi, 2006) Characteristics of physicians who used the Internet were younger than 50, full time or part time academic physicians and males. (Lacher et al., 2000)

Patients are more likely younger and college graduates. Similar to physicians, patients with ethnic minorities are less likely to use emails with their providers. (Ye et al., 2010) In a survey of university based clinics, patients who described themselves as email users were healthier with higher levels of income and education than non email users. (Moyer et al., 2002a)

3.3 Attitudes and barriers to email utilization by physicians and patients

Patients considered email communication with providers as a convenient way of communication that enhances their access to their health care provider and thus improve quality of care. (Ye et al., 2010) Reasons given by email users about their reluctance to send email to their physicians were mainly their lack of knowledge of their physician's email or whether their provider uses email. (Sittig et al., 2001) Other barriers included patient concerns about the effectiveness and efficiency of the email communication. (Moyer et al., 2002a)

Physician's attitudes towards email communication varied among agreement with its potential for enhancing access to patients, restricted use of email communication and adequacy for administrative issues (Moyer et al., 2002b). Important barriers or concerns cited among physicians are lack of time and increase in workload, security and confidentiality, and reimbursement. (Gaster et al., 2003; Moyer et al., 2002b; Pizziferri et al., 2003) However, studies have not proven this fear of increase in workload. Over 6 months period, there was no increase in the volume of messages or time spent answering the messages between physicians who used telephone messages with their patients compared to those who used email communication. (Leong et al., 2005) In university based clinics, the majority of the physicians used email communication with their patients and self-reported an average of 8 emails per month. (Gaster et al., 2003) Controlled trials have shown that physicians respond to an average of 12-13 emails per week spending 5-10 minutes a day. (Virji et al., 2006)

When email users in the general population were asked about their willingness to pay for email communication with their providers, 47% reported that they will not be willing to pay for email communications and 38% were ready to play 5-10 dollars. (Sittig et al., 2001) On the other hand, 42% of patients surveyed in the waiting room of a primary care clinic were willing to pay a small annual fee for this service. (Virji et al., 2006)

Physicians had their concerns about the content of email communications. Physicians do not consider emails suitable for investigation of new symptoms or discussion of mental issues. (Gaster et al., 2003) More than two thirds agree that it is appropriate to communicate with a patient by email about appointment scheduling, medication refills and informing patient about normal results; while half of the physicians only consider disease management and dose adjustment and discussion of abnormal results are appropriate. (Gaster et al., 2003)

Both HIPAA regulations and AMA guidelines emphasize greatly confidentiality and privacy; yet most physicians and patients did not express this concern. Only 20-30% of email users report concern about security or possibility of others reading the email other than their physician as a barrier to email communication between patients and providers. (Sittig et al., 2001; Moyer et al., 2002a) In a qualitative analysis, most of the physicians who used emails with their patients did not get concerned with confidentiality as "long as the patients are comfortable using email". (Patt et al., 2003)

3.4 Content and structure of emails

Emails used by patients, in general, included one single issue or concern at a time (Anand et al., 2005; White et al., 2004) and were concise and medically relevant. (White et al., 2004) Very few patients include sensitive material in their email communication with their provider. (White et al., 2004) Email content included prescription refills, administrative issues, non urgent consultations and checking laboratory results (Couchman et al., 2001; Leong et al., 2005) Content analysis of emails between pediatricians and parents showed that email messages contained one concern at a time with inquiry about a medical question or medical update in the majority of the emails. (Anand et al., 2005) Content analysis of adult email communication with their provider included mainly information updates (42%), followed by prescription renewal and health questions (38%), and inquiry about test results (11%) (White et al., 2004) Though physicians are worried over an increase in workload and the content of emails, around half of the emails sent to the providers were mainly updates and did not require a physician response in 2 studies addressing adult and pediatric population. (Anand et al., 2005; White et al., 2004)

In general population surveys, the expected response time from the physician is between 1-2 days. (Sittig et al., 2001) However, in a study of patients in family practice clinics in central Taxis were more demanding in a very short response time; 21%, 53% and 26% of patients expected a response time to laboratory results in less than 9 hours, 9 to 24 hours and more than 24 hours respectively. (Couchman et al., 2001)

3.5 Ethical and legal concerns

Many argue that the utilization of Emails communication incur an element of injustice among patients who do not have access to the Internet especially the poor and elderly patients. In a study about email use among patients of a primary clinic, patients who reported lack of email access were more likely to be Black or Medicaid insured. (Virji et al., 2006) Moreover, email communication has the potential to improve the care and decrease the workload at the clinic if it was used by elderly patients with multiple comorbidities who frequently utilize the health service. Although 52 (1.3%) out of 4059 patients over 65 years of age reported use of email with their community based physicians, 50% expressed enthusiasm about possibility of using it. (Singh et al., 2009) Jurisdictional issues play an important role if the physician and patients are located in different states or countries. Physicians should be aware of their state/country laws concerning email communications and licensed health actions.

3.6 Benefits of email communication

Email communication between patients and physicians has the potential to improve quality and efficiency of health care. Emails are simple and can be executed at the patient's and physician's convenient time thus eliminating the telephone associated interruptions. It can decrease the unneeded office visits to check normal results or ask for a refill or an administrative issue. Email communications can aid in patient education by attaching relevant documents or referring the patient to reliable internet website. Email use enhances the communication between physicians and patients thus improve satisfaction of patients. In a controlled study, use of emails increased patients' satisfaction in convenience and amount of time spent in their contact with their physician. (Leong et al., 2005) Emails can serve as visit extenders for patients who live in remote places or elderly with limited ability to use transportation means.

3.7 Guidelines of proper use of email communications

Both the American Medical Association (AMA) and American Medical Information Association (AMIA) have established guidelines for proper use of email communications between patients and physicians. (Kane & Sands, 1998; Robertson, 2001) They focus on assurance of proper clear safe communication.

3.7.1 Establishment of expected turnaround time

Establish a document describing the expected turnaround time. Inform the patients not to use emails for urgent issues. Inform the patients about your policies in case of vacation and unavailability.

3.7.2 Establishment of email types and handling

Establish the types of topics that you will discuss through email. Remind the patients not to use emails for sensitive and private issues. Instruct the patient to mention the reason for the consultation in the subject of the email and include his patient identification number in the body of the message. Use autoreply and acknowledge options by patient and yourself to insure the receipt of the emails. Send an email informing the patient of his completed request. Make your statement clear and concise.

3.7.3 Completion of informed consent from patients

Prepare an informed consent that cover all the above items and make sure the patient signs the informed consent and is documented in his medical chart. Include in your informed consent a statement that releases you from liability in case of technical failures.

3.7.4 Documentation in the chart

Print the email communication and insert into the medical chart of the patient. In the presence of electronic medical record, the email should be part of the medical file of the patient.

3.7.5 Assurance of privacy and protection

Use encrypted messages for safe transmission of emails. Inform the patients that emails are not completely safe especially if they use their work emails. Inform the patient if any of your office staff might have access to the emails for triage purposes.

4. Phone communication

The first phone call ever recorded was for a medical need. When Alexander Graham Bell's accidentally spilled battery acid on himself, his famous quote, "Watson, come here I need you" gave birth to the first telephone message and simultaneously to the role of the telephone in medical care. (Car & Sheikh, 2003)

4.1 Scope of mobile phone communications between patients and physicians

Telephone consultations have been widely used in daily activities of clinics in the past few decades and accounts for at least 25% of patient encounters. (Delichatsios et al., 1998) Although use of telephone consultations has increased tremendously, it has been in the context of the clinic setting, triage during after-hours and administrative issues. The access of patients to their own providers through contacting the personal mobile phone of the physician is still in its infancy. Less than half of primary care practitioners reported giving their cell phone number to patients; one third gave their number to only a small percentage of patients. (Peleg et al., 2011)

4.2 Characteristics of mobile phone communications between physicians and patients

There is limited research addressing the magnitude of use of patients of cellular phones to communicate with their physicians. In 2001, a physician recorded his cellular phone calls received from patients over 3 months and found out that he had 94 patient calls; 10% of them occurred during the weekend when the majority occurred during clinic hours at the time he was seeing other patients. Mean duration of calls was 5.8 minutes. They asked about advice on treatment (29%), second opinion (26%), results of medical tests (15%), drug prescription or medical form (12%). (Peleg, 2001)

Characteristics of frequent land telephone callers might be extrapolated to mobile phone use. Characteristic of after hour frequent callers included female gender, frequent office, hospital and emergency room visits. (Hildebrandt et al., 2004) In general, telephone consultations are shorter, include fewer problems, and require less data gathering than face to face consultations. (McKinstry et al., 2010)

4.3 Benefits of mobile phone communication

Potential benefits of telephone consultations are improved access and convenience to patients. (Car & Sheikh, 2003) Mobile phone consultations have the benefit of after hour easy access to the physician overcoming answering machines. Giving mobile phone number to patients gives the impression that the physician is caring and increases the trust relationship between the physician and patient. (Dillaway, 2009) Potential benefits recognized by physicians who provide their cell phone number to patients include reduction of clinic visits, reassuring the patient and giving them a sense of security. (Peleg et al., 2011) Patients reported that they would go to emergency rooms if they were unable to contact a physician. (Delichatsios et al., 1998)

Moreover, after hour call might help reassure patients and improve the triage process. Consider a mother calling for advice concerning a fall of her child with lip lacerations. As a physician, you have no clue about the depth of the laceration and whether it needs emergency transfer for suturing or just reassuring. A cell phone with supported camera can be of utmost benefit in this situation. Majority of patients attending a rural practice in New Zealand showed enthusiasm about using their mobile cameras for medical triage; physicians, as well, were satisfied with the quality of images for diagnosis. (Jayaraman et al., 2008)

4.4 Safety concerns

One of the great challenges of phone consultations is risk of medical errors. A descriptive, retrospective case review of all the telephone-related close malpractice claims showed 3 most common errors categories: poor documentation, faulty triage decisions and incomplete history taking over the phone. (Katz et al., 2008) Using simulated patients, less than one half of resident and attending pediatricians took an adequate history and more than one third made inappropriate management decisions. (Yanovski et al., 1992)

Telephone consultations were judged less likely to include sufficient information to exclude important serious illnesses. (McKinstry et al., 2010) Failing to recognize the potential seriousness of a frustrated patient's multiple calls for the same problem is potential source of medical error because the multiple providers taking the calls were unaware of prior calls. (Katz et al., 2008) In terms of safety, more than 70% of clinicians and 60% of patients were concerned that clinicians would be more likely to make a wrong/inaccurate diagnosis in telephone consultation compared to face-to-face consultations. (McKinstry et al., 2009)

Challenges with telephone consultations include the lack of nonverbal clues, no direct observations and examinations, lack of active listening as the physician might be engaged in his own activities at time of call and talking to family members. Mobile phone cameras and audio recording can have the potential to compensate for the lack of observations.

4.5 Applications of mobile phone telecommunications

mHealth or mobile health is defined as the practice of medicine that is supported by mobile devices such as cellular phones and PDAs. There has been a tremendous improvement in mobile phones technologies, mobile cameras, data processing, network accessibility, and storage capabilities. Mobile phone health related applications target different aspects of health care. Some commercial applications are used by the patient himself for caloric counting, record keeping. Other applications are connected to home based monitoring devices and aid the users to track their vital signs or disease measurements to be shared with their health care provider. Use of mobile phones, in primary care, can be extended to health promotion and awareness campaigns. A short message service (SMS) sending advice and support to smoking cessation among adolescents improved their quit rates at 6 weeks. (Patrick et al., 2008) Participants in an Internet and mobile phone based intervention were provided with wrist worn accelerometer and Bluetooth compatible mobile phone. Weekly exercise plans were offered and email / mobile phone reminders were issued with feedback on their barriers. The intervention motivated healthy adults and significantly increased their level of physical activity. (Hurling et al., 2007) SMS can be used for reminding patients of their health maintenance tests. Mobile phones can be used in self-monitoring chronic diseases and filling diaries. SMS collection of asthma diary data was favored by selectively motivated asthmatic patients due to its integration in their daily life activities as one patient asserted: "...I am not good at routines. Therefore, it is great to get a reminder saying, 'take your medication.' It gives me freedom and creates control." (Anhoj & Moldrup, 2004)

Mobile phone facilitates the interaction between primary care practitioners and specialists especially in remote areas. This improved communication will impact the quality of care delivered to patients. Mobile phones are accessible with the providers at all times which decrease the burden on providers who are in call. They can still enjoy their personal life, though interrupted, while on call and serving patients. The transmission of radiologic pictures using mobile phone multimedia messaging (MMS) was feasible and cost effective for rapid management of musculoskeletal injuries in a remote hospital. (Archbold et al., 2005)

5. Conclusion

Globalization, increased awareness of patients and enthusiasm to control their health and lack of specialists in rural areas will continue to impact the growth and expansion of telemedicine applications in the future. There exist many successful practices of telemedicine in home monitoring and management of chronic diseases, teleconsultation with specialists. Both physicians and patients are willing to increase their communication with each other through email and mobile phones. However, telemedicine has its legal, financial and ethical limitations and challenges that need to be addressed and standardized. Primary care physicians need to be prepared to be technology savvy and change their office settings in order to be able to meet the future demand of telemedicine applications.

6. References

Anand, S. G., Feldman, M. J., Geller, D. S., Bisbee, A., & Bauchner, H. (2005). A content analysis of e-mail communication between primary care providers and parents. *Pediatrics, 115,* 1283-1288.

Anhoj, J. & Moldrup, C. (2004). Feasibility of collecting diary data from asthma patients through mobile phones and SMS (short message service): response rate analysis and focus group evaluation from a pilot study. *J.Med.Internet.Res., 6,* e42.

Archbold, H. A., Guha, A. R., Shyamsundar, S., McBride, S. J., Charlwood, P., & Wray, R. (2005). The use of multi-media messaging in the referral of musculoskeletal limb injuries to a tertiary trauma unit using: a 1-month evaluation. *Injury, 36,* 560-566.

Boodley, C. A. (2006). Primary care telehealth practice. *J.Am.Acad.Nurse Pract., 18,* 343-345.

Bratton, R. L. & Cody, C. (2000). Telemedicine applications in primary care: a geriatric patient pilot project. *Mayo Clin.Proc., 75,* 365-368.

Brooks, R. G. & Menachemi, N. (2006). Physicians' use of email with patients: factors influencing electronic communication and adherence to best practices. *J.Med.Internet.Res., 8,* e2.

Car, J. & Sheikh, A. (2003). Telephone consultations. *BMJ, 326,* 966-969.

Chandhanayingyong, C., Tangtrakulwanich, B., & Kiriratnikom, T. (2007). Teleconsultation for emergency orthopaedic patients using the multimedia messaging service via mobile phones. *J.Telemed.Telecare., 13,* 193-196.

Couchman, G. R., Forjuoh, S. N., & Rascoe, T. G. (2001). E-mail communications in family practice: what do patients expect? *J.Fam.Pract., 50,* 414-418.

Currell, R., Urquhart, C., Wainwright, P., & Lewis, R. (2000). Telemedicine versus face to face patient care: effects on professional practice and health care outcomes. *Cochrane.Database.Syst.Rev.,* CD002098.

Delichatsios, H., Callahan, M., & Charlson, M. (1998). Outcomes of telephone medical care. *J.Gen.Intern.Med., 13,* 579-585.

Dillaway, W. C. (2009). Why I give my cell phone number to my patients. *Fam.Pract.Manag., 16,* 24-25.

Gaster, B., Knight, C. L., DeWitt, D. E., Sheffield, J. V., Assefi, N. P., & Buchwald, D. (2003). Physicians' use of and attitudes toward electronic mail for patient communication. *J.Gen.Intern.Med., 18,* 385-389.

Hildebrandt, D. E., Westfall, J. M., Nicholas, R. A., Smith, P. C., & Stern, J. (2004). Are frequent callers to family physicians high utilizers? *Ann.Fam.Med., 2,* 546-548.

Hurling, R., Catt, M., Boni, M. D., Fairley, B. W., Hurst, T., Murray, P. et al. (2007). Using internet and mobile phone technology to deliver an automated physical activity program: randomized controlled trial. *J.Med.Internet.Res., 9,* e7.

Jayaraman, C., Kennedy, P., Dutu, G., & Lawrenson, R. (2008). Use of mobile phone cameras for after-hours triage in primary care. *J.Telemed.Telecare., 14,* 271-274.

Kane, B. & Sands, D. Z. (1998). Guidelines for the clinical use of electronic mail with patients. The AMIA Internet Working Group, Task Force on Guidelines for the Use of Clinic-Patient Electronic Mail. *J.Am.Med.Inform.Assoc., 5,* 104-111.

Katz, H. P., Kaltsounis, D., Halloran, L., & Mondor, M. (2008). Patient safety and telephone medicine : some lessons from closed claim case review. *J.Gen.Intern.Med., 23,* 517-522.

Kittler, A. F., Carlson, G. L., Harris, C., Lippincott, M., Pizziferri, L., Volk, L. A. et al. (2004). Primary care physician attitudes towards using a secure web-based portal designed to facilitate electronic communication with patients. *Inform.Prim.Care, 12,* 129-138.

Lacher, D., Nelson, E., Bylsma, W., & Spena, R. (2000). Computer use and needs of internists: a survey of members of the American College of Physicians-American Society of Internal Medicine. *Proc.AMIA.Symp.,* 453-456.

Leong, S. L., Gingrich, D., Lewis, P. R., Mauger, D. T., & George, J. H. (2005). Enhancing doctor-patient communication using email: a pilot study. *J.Am.Board Fam.Pract., 18,* 180-188.

McKinstry, B., Hammersley, V., Burton, C., Pinnock, H., Elton, R., Dowell, J. et al. (2010). The quality, safety and content of telephone and face-to-face consultations: a comparative study. *Qual.Saf Health Care, 19,* 298-303.

McKinstry, B., Watson, P., Pinnock, H., Heaney, D., & Sheikh, A. (2009). Telephone consulting in primary care: a triangulated qualitative study of patients and providers. *Br.J.Gen.Pract., 59,* e209-e218.

Menachemi, N., Prickett, C. T., & Brooks, R. G. (2011). The use of physician-patient email: a follow-up examination of adoption and best-practice adherence 2005-2008. *J.Med.Internet.Res., 13,* e23.

Moyer, C. A., Stern, D. T., Dobias, K. S., Cox, D. T., & Katz, S. J. (2002a). Bridging the electronic divide: patient and provider perspectives on e-mail communication in primary care. *Am.J.Manag.Care, 8,* 427-433.

Moyer, C. A., Stern, D. T., Dobias, K. S., Cox, D. T., & Katz, S. J. (2002b). Bridging the electronic divide: patient and provider perspectives on e-mail communication in primary care. *Am.J.Manag.Care, 8,* 427-433.

Pare, G., Jaana, M., & Sicotte, C. (2007). Systematic review of home telemonitoring for chronic diseases: the evidence base. *J.Am.Med.Inform.Assoc., 14,* 269-277.

Pare, G., Moqadem, K., Pineau, G., & St-Hilaire, C. (2010). Clinical effects of home telemonitoring in the context of diabetes, asthma, heart failure and hypertension: a systematic review. *J.Med.Internet.Res., 12,* e21.

Patrick, K., Griswold, W. G., Raab, F., & Intille, S. S. (2008). Health and the mobile phone. *Am.J.Prev.Med., 35,* 177-181.

Patt, M. R., Houston, T. K., Jenckes, M. W., Sands, D. Z., & Ford, D. E. (2003). Doctors who are using e-mail with their patients: a qualitative exploration. *J.Med.Internet.Res., 5,* e9.

Peleg, R. (2001). Off-the-cuff cellular phone consultations in a family practice. *J.R.Soc.Med., 94,* 290-291.

Peleg, R., Avdalimov, A., & Freud, T. (2011). Providing cell phone numbers and email addresses to Patients: the physician's perspective. *BMC.Res.Notes, 4,* 76.

Pizziferri, L., Kittler, A., Volk, L. A., Hobbs, J., Jagannath, Y., Wald, J. S. et al. (2003). Physicians' perceptions toward electronic communication with patients. *AMIA.Annu.Symp.Proc.,* 972.

Robertson, J. (2001). Guidelines for physician-patient electronic communcation. http://www.ama-assn.org/ama/pub/category/2386.html.

Singh, H., Fox, S. A., Petersen, N. J., Shethia, A., & Street, R. L., Jr. (2009). Older patients' enthusiasm to use electronic mail to communicate with their physicians: cross-sectional survey. *J.Med.Internet.Res., 11,* e18.

Sittig, D. F., King, S., & Hazlehurst, B. L. (2001). A survey of patient-provider e-mail communication: what do patients think? *Int J.Med.Inform., 61,* 71-80.

Virji, A., Yarnall, K. S., Krause, K. M., Pollak, K. I., Scannell, M. A., Gradison, M. et al. (2006). Use of email in a family practice setting: opportunities and challenges in patient- and physician-initiated communication. *BMC.Med., 4,* 18.

White, C. B., Moyer, C. A., Stern, D. T., & Katz, S. J. (2004). A content analysis of e-mail communication between patients and their providers: patients get the message. *J.Am.Med.Inform.Assoc., 11,* 260-267.

Yanovski, S. Z., Yanovski, J. A., Malley, J. D., Brown, R. L., & Balaban, D. J. (1992). Telephone triage by primary care physicians. *Pediatrics, 89,* 701-706.

Ye, J., Rust, G., Fry-Johnson, Y., & Strothers, H. (2010). E-mail in patient-provider communication: a systematic review. *Patient.Educ.Couns., 80,* 266-273.

7

Clinical Audit in Primary Care: From Evidence to Practice

Oreste Capelli[1]*, Silvia Riccomi[2], Marina Scarpa[2], Nicola Magrini[3],
Elisabetta Rovatti[4], Imma Cacciapuoti[1] and Antonio Brambilla[1]

[1]*The District Primary Care, Emilia-Romagna Region, Bologna,*
[2]*General Practitioner, Dept of Primary Care, Modena,*
[3]*Drug Evaluation Unit, Emilia-Romagna Health Agency, Bologna,*
[4]*Dept of Pneumology – University Hospital – University of Modena and Reggio Emilia,*
Italy

***Ma anche fra i cultori di scienze, fra i medici pratici, taluni han l'inclinazione
intellettuale a trovare sufficiente qualunque mediocre spiegazione,
mentre altri durano gran fatica ad acquietarsi.*
Augusto MURRI, Professor of Internal Medicine, Bologna University, Italy, 1905.

1. Introduction

The word *Audit* is borrowed from economics and stands for the examination of records or financial accounts with the purpose of checking their accuracy. In a wider sense, an *audit* can be described as an inspection of the accounting procedures and records by a trained accountant, as it happens in business management or information technology (Simon, 2008).

Clinical Audit is a term which has acquired different meanings over time in relation to health care quality. Ten years ago the National Institute for Clinical Excellence (NICE, 2002) published the first manual of Clinical Audit, with the classical definition "Clinical audit is a quality improvement process that seeks to improve patient care and outcomes through systematic review of care against explicit criteria and the implementation of change".

More recently, a new definition has been proposed by the National Clinical Audit Advisory Group (NCAAG, 2010): "Clinical audit is the assessment of the process (using evidence-based criteria) and/or the outcome of care (by comparison with others). Its aim is to stimulate and support national and local quality improvement interventions and, through re-auditing, to assess the impact of such interventions."

The basic requirements to match a well-designed Clinical Audit to clinical praxis are:

---

* Corresponding Author
**Both among scientists and clinical practictioners, some find it easier to rely upon trivial explanations, while others never stop looking for answers.

- changing the usual clinical praxis (care) into the best available practice (**improvement process),**
- basing it on a **systematic review** of knowledge and praxis,
- conducting it with **explicit criteria**, sustained by evidence based knowledge and with **measurable end-points** (indicators),
- completing it with an **implementation pathway**, putting knowledge into praxis.

Further, and not less important, benefits are connected with a good clinical audit: opportunities for education and training, easier relationships among clinicians, clinical teams, managers and patients, improvements in service delivery and patient outcomes (NHS Wirral, 2012).

2. Clinical Audit in Primary Care (PC): What it is and what it isn't

(Quality) is the point at which subject and object meet…. Quality is not a thing. It is an event…. It is the event at which the subject becomes aware of the object. (Pirsig, 1974)***

2.1 Audit and Clinical Governance

In the last 40 years, a dramatic evolution in healthcare protection has taken place, starting a race towards the sustainable effectiveness of health procedures. Managers and directors have mainly focused on the economic aspects of healthcare, planning therefore all activities in terms of availability of resources. Later on, more and more importance was given to the quality of care, where effectiveness was to be associated with appropriateness, safety, fair and equal participation of every individual user. All these characteristics concur to the Clinical Governance (CG) of a healthcare system.

The CG is "a system through which healthcare organisations are accountable for continuously improving the quality of their services and safeguarding high standards of care by creating an environment in which excellence in clinical care will flourish" (Scally & Donaldson, 1998). The CG is also a system centred on the patient's needs. Effective involvement of both patients and carers is essential in order to attain the main target of quality of care. (Zwanenberg & Harrison, 2004). The CG is not just a new organizing facility, but the very core of a health policy based on the quality of care, through strong interactions among its multiple components (Table 1), as reported by Starey (Starey, 2001). Clinical Audit is an essential and integral part of CG (Burgess, 2011; Zwanenberg & Harrison, 2004; Wienand, 2009).

2.2 What is Clinical Audit (in Primary Care)

"Audit & feedback" continues to be widely used as a strategy to improve professional practice. Healthcare professionals should be obviously prompted to modify their practice once they are given feedback that their clinical practice is inconsistent with that of their peers or accepted guidelines. A Cochrane systematic review (Jamtvedt et al, 2006), evaluated

---

***Pirsig Robert M. (1974) "Zen and the Art of Motorcycle Maintenance" Publisher: William Morrow & Company, first edition, ISBN 0-688-00230-7.

118 clinical trials to assess the effects of audit and feedback on healthcare professionals' practice, and patients' outcomes. Jamtvedt et al. conclude that their effects on the improvement of professional practice are generally modest to moderate. The effectiveness of "Audit & feedback" is likely to be greater when baseline adherence to recommended practice is low and when feedback is delivered more intensively.

Clinical Audit has been more extensively applied in secondary care, where the majority of the scientific literature comes from. Since the role of the PC is being considered by all healthcare policy makers as an increasingly important part of future healthcare provision, clinical audit should be applied to this level of practice in order to assess whether patients are receiving the best quality of care (Burgess, 2011). A fundamental part of a good practice implies regular monitoring of standards of care and the willingness to make changes. Measuring the practice through Clinical Audit provides the best available tool to know when change is needed. (Benjamin, 2008).

- Participation of all professionals in Clinical Audit;
- Evidence-based practice is supported and applied routinely in everyday practice, use of guidelines and implementation of recommendations;
- Effective monitoring of clinical care with high quality systems for clinical record keeping, the collection of relevant information and assessing outcomes;
- Clinical risk systematically assessed with programmes in place to reduce risk
- Critical incident reporting ensures that adverse events are identified, openly investigated, lessons are learned and promptly applied
- Complaints procedures accessible to patients and their families
- Involvement of patients and their families
- Education and training
- Research and development

Table 1. Elements of Clinical Governance (CG) (adapted from Starey, 2001)

According to Benjamin (2008), there are several elements (or tools) to perform an effective Clinical Audit in PC:

- The audit should be part of a structured programme and should have a local leader;
- Clinical audit should assess structure, process, or outcomes of care;
- Audit should ideally be multidisciplinary;
- Patients should ideally be part of the audit;
- Audit topics should be chosen in relation to high risk, high volume, or high cost problems or in relation to national clinical audits;
- Standards should be selected from good quality guidelines;
- Action plans should be devised so as to overcome the local obstacles to changes, and to identify the right people for service improvement;
- Audits should be repeated in order to find out whether improvements in care have been implemented as a result of a previous cycle;
- Specific mechanisms and systems should be developed to monitor and reinforce service improvements once the audit cycle has been completed.

Clinical Audit in PC should be part of the ordinary working procedures, where professionals share and compare their daily activity with evidence-based standards adapted to fit their settings. However, clinical practice in PC is hard and complex and can seldom be assessed by means of a linear cause-effect approach: too many ungovernable and unpredictable events occur between a physician's prescription and a clinical outcome, i.e. understanding of information, patient's compliance, drugs tolerability, facilities presence or absence in the local healthcare system, etc. Other obstacles may be found in the very habits, attitudes and motivations of the professionals themselves (see paragraph 3.4 on audit barriers). Since the outcome is never guaranteed, that is the main reason why, at the end of any process, a re-assessment of the performance is needed.

2.3 What Clinical Audit is not (in Primary Care)

"Research is concerned with discovering the right thing to do;
Audit with ensuring that it is done right "(Smith R, 1992)

Clinical Audit in PC is neither a case report discussion, nor a way of managing healthcare resources, though its results can give useful suggestions in this direction. Furthermore, Clinical Audit is not simply a means of producing data and statistics, especially with control purposes. Finally, Clinical Audit is not a synonym for research: it aims to assess to what extent a process is consistent with best practice and/or achieves expected outcomes.

Research helps to answer the question *'What is best practice?'*. It is concerned with creating new knowledge about which treatment works better in a given clinical situation. It lays the foundations of consensus about the type of care that we should be providing. Clinical Audit answers the question, *'Are we following agreed best practice?'*. However, research and audit are closely linked. Without research, it is impossible to know what best practice actually is; without audit, it is impossible to know whether we are following best practice (Simon, 2008). Both research and clinical audit may involve measurement of patient outcomes, even though their purpose is different: if the objectives are clear, one should concentrate on three questions:

1. Is the purpose of your project to try and improve the quality of patient care?	Yes	No
2. Will the project involve measuring current practice against standards?	Yes	No
3. Does the project include anything being done to patients beyond their routine clinical management?	Yes	No

If the answers are 'yes' to the first two questions and 'no' to the third, the project is very likely to fall within the remit of clinical audit (Potter et al, 2010).

Research and Clinical Audit are distinct activities with different goals (table 2).

However, Audit and Research are interrelated in four ways (Black, 1992):

- Clinical Audit can provide high-quality data for non-experimental evaluative research;
- Research provides a basis for defining good-quality care for audit purposes;
- Research into the effectiveness and cost-effectiveness of clinical audit is essential in order to establish the value of different interventions;
- Research is to be audited in order to ensure that high-quality work is performed.

	Clinical Audit	Observational Research	Experimental Research
Purpose	To evaluate how closely local practice resembles best practice.	To formulate questions on a theme relating to practice or policy	To establish the best or most effective practice.
Questions	Are we doing the right thing? Are we actually doing what we think we are doing?	What happens about this thing under the present circumstances?	What is the right thing to be done?
Knowledge	It provides knowledge primarily about the service being audited.	It provides knowledge primarily about the relationship between an event and its (possible) cause/s	It aims to add new knowledge to the large body of published research knowledge.
Methods	No allocation to treatment groups; final results should be influenced by auditors who identify areas of non-conformity with evidence-based practice and apply changing strategies before re-audit	Clear sampling methods, with reasonable response rate (>40%); final results shouldn't be influenced by researchers' intervention	Pre-specified research plans together with hypotheses related to the objective of the intervention; final results shouldn't be influenced by researchers' judgement
Sample size	The number of cases, based on previous findings, should be large enough to influence practice	The size should be sufficiently large to avoid sampling bias, so that surveys can have wide applicability	Statistically supported sample size (depending on expected effect)
Data analysis	Simple statistics (e.g. means, frequencies) to compare audit cycles	Simple descriptive statistics	Data analyses are required for inference making
Results compared	with standards that define good practice.	with a cohort of not exposed subjects	with a randomized control group
Implications of results	The results mostly have implications for the service being audited.	The results mainly have implications for specific populations and context	The results have implications for the whole field of health-care and often beyond it.
Reports	Results are often only reported locally and the identity of clinicians is protected.	Results are reported publicly and the researcher is open to scrutiny.	Results are reported publicly and the researcher is open to scrutiny.
Ethical approval	Not required	Often not required	Always required
Outcome	Strategies in place to improve clinical practice	Leading to clinical effectiveness strategy (e.g. guidance or audit)	Improved basic or/and applied knowledge

	Clinical Audit	Observational Research	Experimental Research
Afterwards	Practice changes, then the audit is repeated in the same way to see if the changes obtain the desired effect.	The research may be repeated with different populations or in different contexts to expand the knowledge about causes and effects	Other people will repeat the research to test or add to the validity of the result, or to challenge the hypothesis.

Table 2. Similarities and differences among Clinical Audit and Research (Observational or Experimental) – modified and integrated from Brain et al, 2009; Clark & Rowe, 2002; and Potter et al, 2010.

3. How to conduct a Clinical Audit: The circular pathway (Audit cycle)

Good preparation is crucial to the success of a clinical audit project. Topic choice will be determined by a number of factors, but the focus should be one of identifying opportunities for improving care. Clinical audit involves looking at one's own practice, not that of others, but the priorities of those receiving care can differ quite markedly from the priorities of those giving care. User involvement is therefore fundamental to successful, meaningful audit. For this reason stakeholders need to be involved in the process at all stages, appropriately using their skills in and knowledge of the audit topic. All those involved in audit need access to training and/or advice in conducting audit projects to develop their skills and to ensure the effectiveness of projects undertaken (Burgess, 2011).

Clinical audits are best conducted within a structured program, adequately funded, with clearly defined roles, effective leadership to drive the process, participation by all relevant staff, and an emphasis on team working and support. A timetable to maintain momentum is also essential. Protected time needs to be made available to those involved in audit work if its aim is to achieve improving quality in healthcare (Burgess, 2011).

Clinical audit can be described as a cycle or a spiral (see Figure 1), formed by the succession of determined steps or stages that follow:

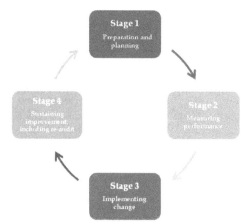

1. a systematic process of establishing best practice,
2. measuring care against criteria,
3. taking action to improve care,
4. and monitoring to sustain improvement.

Fig. 1. The cycle of AUDIT - essential steps (modified from Burgess, 2011).

Questions about clinical praxis Bhopal & Thomson, 1991	NICE, 2002	Actions (Stages) to answer the questions (to implement change of the praxis)
What do we do? What should we do?	*What are we trying to achieve?*	**Stage 1:** preparation, planning and organisation of clinical audit
Do we do what we think we do? Are we doing what we should be doing?	*Are we achieving it?*	**Stage 2:** measuring level of performance (and comparing it with standards)
How can we improve what we do?	*Why are we not achieving it?*	**Stage 3:** making improvements (after analyzing the barriers to change)
Can we improve?	*Have we made things better?*	**Stage 4:** sustaining improvements (after ... ... and ...)

Table 3. Clinical audit answers to some questions with a step-by-step process.

The spiral suggests that as the process continues, each cycle aspires to a higher level of quality (NICE, 2002), to drive up standards of healthcare and service provision (Burgess, 2011). To maintain adherence to the praxis, different questions must find answers in the corresponding steps of the "Audit cycle" (Table 3).

3.1 Clinical Audit: First of all be clear with terms

In clinical audit, criteria , indicators and standards are used to assess a wide range of aspects of the quality of care provided by an individual, a team or an organisation.

Before studying the single steps of the "Audit cycle" we need to focus on the use of some terms that may be either used as synonyms or with different meanings.

Recommendation: it represents the "best practice", as it answers the following question: *"which is the right thing to do (or the worst thing to keep from doing)?"*. Choosing a recommendation for an Audit should come from reviewing and comparing existing Guidelines (GLs) (Baker & Fraser, 1995) in order to enhance the transferability of evidence to different settings (see paragraph 3.2).

Criterion: it is a term used when a recommendation goes from general to specific, measurable and contextualized. It answers the question *"What is the right thing to do for this particular patients in the present situation?"*. Audit criteria are clearly defined, measurable, explicit statements of what should be done to patients, and whenever possible it should be based on up-to-date evidence (Burgess, 2011). There should be adequate research evidence that the recommendations from which they are derived are related to clinical effectiveness, safety and efficiency (Wollersheim et al, 2007). Some examples are outlined in the Quality and Outcomes Framework 2010/11 of the English NHS (QOF, 2012).

Indicator: it is the qualitative and quantitative measure to determine the distance between practice and its standard (Hermens, 2011). Indicators should be explicitly defined as measurable elements of practice performance, for which there is evidence or consensus that they can be used to assess the quality of care. They should therefore change the quality of patient care, clinical support services, and organisational function that affect patient outcomes (CCHSA, 1996; Lawrence 1997). An indicator usually is a mathematical function sometimes measuring the ratio between a number of subjects fulfilling the criterion and the general population, sometimes referring to mean values (e.g. scores at a questionnaire or at a validated scale) (Hermens, 2011). Indicators come from data obtained in field research and therefore depend upon its completeness and precision. In 1966 Donabedian distinguished 3 types of indicators: structure, process and outcome (Table 4).

What indicators measure?	Questions…	…and Answers (with some examples)
The **structure** of care	*What do you need?*	**Staff and resources that enable healthcare:** eg. resources such as the presence of a dedicated stroke unit or a diagnostic facility;
The **process** of care	*What do you do?*	**Investigations, treatments, procedures:** eg. waiting times in clinics, or number of diagnostic procedures performed;
The **outcome** of care	*What do you expect?*	**Measurable change in health status:** eg. reduction of blood pressure or the number of hospital admissions in response to therapy.

Table 4. Indicators in Clinical Audit: some examples..

Many examples of all three types of indicators in the Primary Care setting are outlined in the Quality and Outcomes Framework 2010/11 (QOF, 2012).

Standard: it represents the optimal level of performance. It is the value a specific indicator should have, had the criterion been applied in optimal conditions, eluding known exceptions (e.g.: asthmatic patients with an acute myocardial infarction should not receive beta-blockers). Standards are quantifiable statements detailing the specific aspects of patient care and management that one intends to measure current practice against. According to Bristol Clinical Audit Team standards should be **SMART: S**pecific, **M**easurable, **A**greed, **R**elevant and **T**heoretically sound (UHBristol NHS, 2009).

Standards should always be based on the strongest up-to-date evidence of what constitutes best practice, possibly based on the most widely applicable GLs available. If GLs/protocols do not exist, or existing ones are out of date, it is necessary to undertake a systematic literature search to identify current best practice. Before Clinical Audit starts, on-the-spot agreement on standards is essential. It is hard to improve practice if there is disagreement as to what constitutes best practice.

However according to Anderson in his "ABC of Audit" (2012) there are several types of standard:

a **minimum standard** describes the lowest acceptable standard of performance; minimum standards are often used to distinguish between acceptable and unacceptable practice;

an **ideal standard** describes the care that should be possible to give under ideal conditions, with no constraints. By definition such a standard cannot usually be attained;

an **optimum standard** lies between the minimum and the ideal. Setting an optimum standard requires judgement, discussion and consensus with other members of the team; optimum standards represent the standard of care most likely to be achieved under normal conditions of practice.

Acceptable Performance Level (APL): Performance levels, expressed as a percentage of the standard, should be agreed at the outset of the audit for each audit criterion. They are a compromise between clinical importance, practicability and acceptability (Crombie et al, 1993). APL overlaps Anderson's "minimum standard" (Anderson, 2012) and represents the objective difficulty of transferring ideal criteria (coming from controlled studies) to the real settings. Selecting and developing appropriate performance levels is the core of audit. It is generally agreed that each audit criterion should have a performance level or target assigned to it. Indeed, failure to do this can lead to missed opportunities for improvement, even where practice appears to be good. Open discussion among the audit team members and relevant stakeholders needs to take place in order to agree on the most appropriate performance levels. These are necessary to determine to what degree the audit criteria should be achieved, and to identify whether or not change needs to be implemented (Burgess, 2011).

Benchmark: it is the best real value for a definite indicator; in other words, the best existing performance to which a comparison can be done. It is not always easy to compare results coming from different contexts (geographical, ethnic, cultural), therefore benchmarks must be the best performance of a specific context, referring to settings homogeneous enough to neglect possible discrepancies.

3.2 Stage 1 of the Audit cycle: Preparation, organisation and planning

What do we do? What should we do?
What are we trying to achieve?

The impact of a local audit will be maximized if the topic is relevant to the health system and is likely to improve care delivery; if not only the management is involved, but there is also the involvement of a committed and supportive team, with a committed opinion leader. Furthermore the methodology should be robust, with a limited number of recommendations to be implemented, that identify specific actions, and results presented in a simple, clear manner. A clear plan for improvement needs to be defined since the beginning (Potter et al, 2010).

Choosing a topic. Clinical Audit is a complex time-consuming process. In order to ensure that the audit may also be meaningful to the clinicians involved, it is essential to select an appropriate topic. In Table 5 some questions are reported that may be a useful guide for discussion about prioritizing clinical topics (Potter et al, 2010).

The multiprofessional team has an important role in prioritising clinical topics. The same questions can emerge both from clinicians' offices and from the administrators' desks, but it's clear enough that the objectives might be quite different. Usually, audits are carried out if a service improvement can be achieved, as it is neither effortless nor unexpensive in terms of time and costs.

A project that lacks clear objectives cannot achieve significant goals, so a clear sense of purpose must be established before appropriate methods for audit being considered. Therefore once the clinical audit topic has been agreed upon, the reason(s) for the project must be clearly defined. In team audits this ensures that everyone involved in the audit is working to a common purpose in order that a suitable audit method can be chosen. A discussion on the nature of the problem, first highlighting the need for the audit, is beneficial to ensure clarity of purpose, since there is no guarantee that everyone involved clearly understands the reason(s) for undertaking the audit (Burgess, 2011).

- Is the topic related to high costs, volumes or risks to staff or users?
- Is there any evidence of a serious quality problem (e.g. patients' complaints, high complication rates)?
- Is there strong evidence available to inform standards (e.g. systematic reviews or national clinical guidelines)?
- Is the problem amenable to change?
- Is a sustainable improvement possible?
- Is there any potential for involvement in a national audit project?
- Is the topic pertinent to national policy initiatives?
- Is the topic a priority for the organisation?

Table 5. Main questions for prioritising clinical topics (modified from Potter et al, 2010)

Selecting recommendation(s) and criteria. After choosing the topic for the clinical audit (*What do we do?*), it is necessary to define which one is the best clinical practice (*What should we do?*) and what aims the clinical audit pursues (*What are we trying to achieve?*). With regard to that, great attention must be given in choosing the recommendations (best practice) that lead to criteria and standards (*What should we do?*). Choice of recommendations to be implemented will be more and more accurate with a better definition of the clinical issue.

In 2006, Brown et al. (BMJ) proposed the EPICOT scheme (**E**vidence, **P**opulation, **I**ntervention, **C**omparison, **O**utcome(s) and **T**ime), in order to help researcher address appropriate questions about grey areas lacking clear evidence. Viceversa, in the Clinical Audit, topics should come from areas where strong evidence already exists (see paragraph 2.3), so that the clinical question, sectioned in PICOT fractions, helps choose the best "Evidence" (as "recommendations") for the chosen topic. The complete acronym will become PICOTE. In table 6 a practical example is reported.

Applying the PICOTE scheme to the topic of the Clinical Audit helps define the main points to be examined by means of the audit itself: population, intervention, indicators, outcomes, timing, etc. (see also the Planning Data Collection paragraph).

There should be adequate research evidence that the chosen recommendations are related to clinical effectiveness, safety and efficiency. The information required can be derived by using systematic or non-systematic methods. Non-systematic methods, such as case studies, play an important role in comparing experiences, but they do not tap into available evidence. Systematic methods can be based directly on scientific evidence by combining the best available evidence with expert opinion, or they can be based on clinical guidelines (Wollersheim et al, 2007).

Topic to be audited: **How many people with stable severe COPD who receive an antibiotic prescription to prevent or treat an acute exacerbation of COPD (AECOPD) have been admitted to the hospital?**

What is the Population interested by this topic?	P	All COPD patients with a severe degree of disease (FEV1 less than 50%)
Which Intervention would we like to improve?	I	An antibiotic treatment (to be defined) to prevent/treat an AECOPD
Is there an alternative intervention (Comparison) we would like to consider?	C	An alternative treatment (e.g. another antibiotic, or an oral course of steroids, to be defined) to prevent/treat an AECOPD
On the basis of which Outcomes should we evaluate the effectiveness of I or C?	O	hospital admission or death; antibiotic or steroid course of therapy for each patient; type of antibiotic more used; number of visits for AECOPD; etc.
What is the Time necessary for a complete observation of the topic?	T	e.g. One year (or more or less)
What is the Evidence about this topic? (the more recent and robust)	E	*Recommendation from NICE COPD GLs (2010) :* Giving people at risk of exacerbations a course of antibiotic and corticosteroid tablets ready for use at home. Monitoring the use of these drugs and advising people to contact a healthcare professional if their symptoms do not improve.

Table 6. An example of the PICOTE scheme application to an Audit in General Practice.

Sources of possible evidence-based audit criteria are (Burgess, 2011):

- *Recommendations derived from evidence-based guidelines*: when contextualized in the local setting, they establish the standard (Best Practice) with which to compare the current practice.
- Where there is no national or local guidance available, a literature search *of specific journals* or good-quality *systematic reviews* can be undertaken to identify the best and most up-to-date evidence that can be used to generate audit criteria.
- Sometimes it may be necessary for a *group of professionals* to formulate their own criteria where national guidance or evidence-based literature are not available, and here the use of formal *consensus methods* is preferable.

A greater number of opportunities is now available to work *collaboratively with users (doctors or patients)* in the choice of appropriate and relevant audit criteria. Users can bring a different perspective to those aspects of the verification they consider important to measure.

Establishing acceptable standards (see also paragraph 3.1). Since standards represent audit targets, by which the entity of quality improvement is measured (and often incentivated!) it is very important to pay attention to some "more relational, less technical" aspects (Burgess, 2011), as:

- Who has been consulted about the proposed standards?
- How have standards been selected and agreed upon ?
- Are the standards defined clearly and understood by all?
- If national standards are to be used, do they need to be tailored to local circumstances? (see the Acceptable Performance Level (APL) in paragraph 3.1)
- Do the standards support the ethos of continuous quality improvement by providing a target over and above current practice? (see more in paragraph 7)

Planning Data Collection. A critical issue for audit in General Practice is data collection. It is not a problem of good/bad recording electronic systems, but of data entering. The GPs are often very busy, thus they have difficulties in inserting data properly. Yet, the validity of the data is dependent on the care that is taken to enter data into the records, therefore in some occasions data recording may be useless. The data may be available in a computerised information system, but it may also be appropriate to collect data manually, depending on the outcome being measured (e.g. a questionnaire). In either case, one will need to consider what data he needs to collect, where he will find the data, and who will collect them.

To make sure that the data collected are precise, and that only essential data are collected, certain details about what is to be audited must be established from the outset, like the user group to be included, the healthcare professionals involved in the users' care and the time period over which the criteria apply (NICE, 2002).

According to Burgess (Burgess, 2011), when planning data collection, in order to ensure the effectiveness of a process, it is important to check a list of questions:

- What type of data do I need to collect (quantitative and/or qualitative)?
- What data items will need to be used to show whether or not performance levels have been met for each standard?
- What data sources will be used to find the data?
- Will a data collection tool need to be designed?
- Will I need to collect data prospectively and/or retrospectively?
- What size is the target population and will I need to take a sample?
- How will data be collected (manually and/or electronically)?
- How long will it take to collect the required amount of data?
- Who will be collecting the data?

Finally the population to be audited should be clearly defined, the data required should be made readily and reliably accessible and the measures to be assessed should be meaningful (Burgess,2011).

The sample dimension should be wide enough to be representative of the local clinical practice, but not too wide to make the sample evaluation impossible or too expensive. On the other hand, as Quality and Outcomes Framework 2010/11 shows, a constant monitoring of health quality indicators of a whole population is possible (QOF, 2012).

3.3 Stage 2 of the Audit cycle: Measuring levels of performance

Do we do what we think we do?
Are we doing what we should be doing?
Are we achieving it?

Once the criteria have been defined, we must choose the proper indicators to answer the question *Do we do what we think we do?* As one can see in paragraph 3.1, an indicator is the (quantitative and/or qualitative) measure of the distance between practice and standard Hermens, 2011). Here we can find the answer to the question: *Are we doing what we should be doing? Are we achieving it?*. The characteristics of the indicators that guarantee the quality and pragmatism of an Audit are listed in Table 7.

As mentioned indicators and field data are not synonyms. The latter are essential for the construction of the former.

Although clinical records are frequently used as the source of data, they are often incomplete. Electronic Information Systems (EISs) are useful not only for collecting data but also for improving access to research evidence, prompting change through record templates, and introducing revised systems of care (Benjamin, 2008). Unfortunately in many countries, with very advanced care plan (like Canada and the U.S.), there is lack of performance data from the Primary Care because of the non-use of Electronic Medical Records (EMRs) by GPs. (Hogg & Dyke, 2011).

Relevancy	Relevant to important aspects (effectiveness, safety and efficiency) and dimensions (professional, organisational and patient oriented) of quality of care
Validity	Strong correlation with the current quality of care Valid on the basis of good scientific proof and experience
Reliability	Low inter- and intra-observer variation Available and reliable data sources Statistically reliable, i.e. reported as an average or median with confidence intervals and valid for comparison, i.e. corrected for case mix and socio-demographic variables
Feasibility	Easily available Applicable to quality improvement; i.e. easy to build in improvement initiatives Sensitive to improvement in time Useful to base decisions on caregivers, patients, regulating agencies In relation to those who should use them

Table 7. The quality characteristics of the indicators (modified from Wollersheim et al, 2007)

The audit data can be quantitative (numerical data that can be counted in order to determine whether or not performance levels have been achieved), or qualitative data (concerned with words rather than with numbers).

A qualitative data collection may include descriptive elements, such as additional comments within questionnaire, interviews, narrative based medicine, focus groups and analysis of documents. In some cases a single method may be used while in others a combination of methods may be employed. The emphasis in qualitative research on understanding meanings and experiences makes it particularly useful for quality assessment. If data are to be collected qualitatively, it is advantageous to consult appropriate publications, and to enlist the support of audit staff or others with skills in designing qualitative data collection tools (Burgess, 2011; Pope et al, 2000).

The following key questions need to be asked when determining which method will be used (Burgess, 2011):

-    How are the data stored?
-    Where are the data stored?
-    Who will be collecting the data?
-    Where will the data be collected?
-    Are data being collected retrospectively or prospectively?

Retrospective audit increases the possibility of identifying all patients meeting the inclusion criteria, e.g. complete patient numbers. However it does depend on being able to identify patients through coding or other record systems which fit the inclusion criteria.

Prospective audit increases the chance of good quality data collection, but there is the risk that some patients, in particular those who it might be important to audit, will be missed and there will be incomplete patient numbers. Furthermore there is a risk that, because teams are aware that an audit is on-going, clinical practice may be altered. In some ways this is a good thing if it means patients get better care, but it may result in a false evaluation of routine care. (HQIP, 2009).

Data collection can be implemented both by in- or out-personnel, with a good knowledge of the clinical process and of the data they have to pick up and specifically trained in working with survey instruments.

Data analysis can be performed with different methods, from the simplest (percentages, quotients) to the most sophisticated statistical techniques. In the majority of cases, simpler methods are preferable, as any of the personnel can easily understand them and what they mean. In this line, it is essential to complete data analysis with easily understandable reports, where differences with standard values, and both positive and negative results must be clearly shown. If the discussion on how well the standards were met generates the answer "quite good" the audit could stop, or the objectives may be changed (for example, changing levels of APL); but if the standards were not met, an analysis of the reasons for the divergent results (Stage 3) and a plan on how to make improvements are recommended.

3.4 Stage 3 of the Audit cycle: Implementing change, making improvements

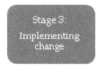

How can we improve what we do?
Why are we not achieving it?

To improve current clinical practice, it is necessary to find the causes of suboptimal performances *(Why are we not achieving it?)*, i.e. low resources, professionals' or patients' characteristics. If a cause can be detected (*What are the barriers to change?*), a shorter way to its solution is at hand (*How can we improve what we do?*).

Clinical audit is a structured change process. All audit projects must include a programme of change activity and post- identification of the findings from audit (re-audit), to ensure that necessary changes will happen. An accurate planning for implementation is probably the most important element for the implementation of change (Burgess, 2011).

Implementing change. Implementing new knowledge into practice requires deliberate and planned effort. Implement knowledge is "the scientific study of methods to promote the systematic uptake of research findings and other evidence-based practices into routine practice, and, hence, to improve the quality and effectiveness of health services". It includes the study of influences on healthcare professional and organisational behaviour. (Eccles & Miiman, 2006).

Grol and Grimshaw emphasizes the need for an implementation plan. There should be a good basis for change: this could be either new scientific knowledge, or perhaps the identification of a particular practice problem or of a best practice. Afterwards, the implementation should be planned: **when, where, how, and by whom the implementation will occur.** An in-depth analysis can reveal the target group and behaviours, and identify barriers and facilitators to change. The general principles of planning are similar across different projects and circumstances. They include plan development, testing, adapting and scheduling, and evaluation and organisation of the implementation (Grol et al, 2005).

It may be helpful to undertake a diagnostic analysis to identify factors that will influence the likelihood of change before selecting the most appropriate strategies and interventions for implementing change. The Healthcare Quality Improvement Partnership (Schofield & Jenkins, 2009) has recently released useful examples for a pragmatic approach to a plan of implementation (Table 8).

Barriers to change. Most theories on implementation of evidence in health care emphasize the importance of developing a good understanding of possible barriers to change, in order to develop an effective intervention (Grol, 1997). Whether considered in the context of models for quality and safety improvement or guideline implementation initiatives (Ashford et al 1999; Grol et al,2005; Lomas, 1994; Robertson et al, 1996), systematic reviews of improvement interventions (Chaillet et al, 2006; Grimshaw et al, 2004) or guideline adoption (Cabana et al, 1999), barriers are believed to influence the success of improvement strategies in a very important way.

A recent Cochrane Review analyzed 26 studies to assess the effectiveness of interventions tailored to identify barriers to change on professional practice or patient outcomes. Authors' conclusions stated that interventions tailored to prospectively identified barriers are more likely to improve professional practice than no intervention or the simple dissemination of guidelines (Baker et al, 2010).

Barriers to change have been classified by the Cochrane Effective Practice and Organisation of Care Group (EPOC, 2002) into nine categories: information management, clinical uncertainty, sense of competence, perceptions of liability, patient expectations, standards of practice, financial disincentives, administrative constraints and other.

The barriers can act at individual, team or organisation levels (Ferlie & Shortell, 2001; Garside, 1998). The possible barriers to a plan of implementation should be identified by means of (Burgess, 2011):

- interviews with key staff and/or users;
- discussion at a team meeting;
- observations of patterns of work;
- identification of the care pathway;
- facilitated team meetings, with the use of brainstorming or fishbone diagrams.

Step	General objective	Specific actions
1	Enlist the support and involvement of key people	Identify key stakeholders and ensure that they are involved and their contribution is valued. Use the stakeholder team as agents of change across the wider organisation(s) and try to achieve a good mix of skills, authority, resources and leadership.
2	Develop a clear project plan	Create a simple plan for life span of the project, which clearly defines roles and responsibilities. Get people involved in the plan, especially if they are directly affected by it. Make sure that the plan is built in small, achievable chunks with realistic timescales.
3	Support the plan with consistent behaviours	Whatever the characteristics of the change are, either cost-cutting, behavioural, or ways of working, it is important to be seen to be "walking the talk". People are only likely to adopt change if it is demonstrated by all levels (and particularly senior levels) of the organisation
4	Develop "enabling structures"	Recognise what needs to happen to support the change. Training workshops, communication sessions, team meetings that are aligned to the change will help people understand the reasons for the change, and buy-in to the process.
5	Celebrate milestones	When milestones are achieved, celebrate the fact that progress has been made. Recognising progress will maintain motivation and stakeholder interest, and give confidence that the longer term vision is achievable.
6	Communicate relentlessly	This is probably the most important activity of all. Communicating effectively can motivate, overcome resistance, lay out the pros and cons of change, and give employees a stake in the process.

Table 8. The Six Steps for Implementing Change (adapted from Schofield & Jenkins, 2009)

To understand and plan tailored strategies to overcome the barriers (Table 9) are critical step for the improvement process (Grol & Grimshaw, 2003). The greatest barrier to change is the attitude that nothing can be done. It should be part of the professional practice of all doctors to be continually asking themselves: *"How could we be doing this better?"*. Having asked the question, they should think carefully how things could be done differently and consider with colleagues how to improve care. However, many do manage to improve services. To counteract the barriers in order to realize a Clinical Audit in Primary Care, it is necessary to stress and reinforce the already existing positive factors (Table 10).

Changes in care are not always associated with increasing costs: significant efficiency and cost saving can coexist with improved quality (Potter et al, 2010).

Making improvements. Audit is concerned with improving care, and an action plan should be developed to improve either the structure or process of care as this should lead to an improvement in outcome (Copeland, 2005).

When it has been agreed what changes are needed, it is necessary to implement those changes. Depending on the changes, it may be necessary to alter individuals' roles and responsibilities to do this, and staff training may be necessary (Bristol NHS, 2009).

Practitioners need to consider what is the best way to feedback the results from their audit. Potential stages for dissemination include team meetings, departmental newsletters, local clinical audit meetings, professional development meetings. Results will generally include recommendations for improvement, which may relate to clinical practice or administration procedures. Any changes proposed as a consequence of the audit should be shared and developed with staff affected. Steps towards change should be identified, a timescale agreed and tasks for individuals decided. Implementing recommendations forms the more difficult part of the audit cycle (M.E.R.G., 2012).

In Figure 2 an example of activity planning from a Clinical Audit on Chronic Obstructive Pulmonary Disease (COPD)is reported. The principal objective was the improvement of diagnosis, severity classification and inhalatory therapy in COPD patients in a District in Northern Italy. Both General Practitioners and Hospital Specialists were involved.

	Potential barriers	Examples of barriers
Practice environment (organisational context)	Financial disincentives	Lack of reimbursement
	Organisational constraints	Lack of time
	Perception of liability	Risk of formal complaint
	Patient's expectations	Expressed wishes related to prescription
Prevailing opinion (social context)	Standards of practice	Usual routines
	Opinion leaders	Key persons not agreeing with evidence
	Medical training	Obsolete knowledge
	Advocacy	Advocacy by pharmaceutical companies
Knowledge and attitudes (professional context)	Clinical uncertainty	Unnecessary test for vague symptoms
	Sense of competence	Self confidence in skills
	Compulsion to act	Need to do something
	Information overload	Inability to appraise evidence

Table 9. Example of barriers to implementation of evidence (modified from Grol & Grimshaw, 2003).

Audit Stage	Activity	2005				2006			
		March - May	May - July	September - October	November - December	January - June	July - August	September - October	December
Stage 1	Appointment of multidisciplinary team	■							
	Selection of the recommendations and definition of standards and indicators	■							
	Writing Audit protocol and planning data collection		■						
	Clinical Audit accreditation for CME		■						
	Recruitment of GPs		■						
	Presentation of Protocol to GPs and Hospital specialist in the District		■						
Stage 2	Basal Data collection (from GPs and hospital specialists)			■					
	Data Analysis and Assessment of the gap between results and standards								
Stage 3	Evaluation of the results and Analysis of the Barriers				■				
	Educational Interventions (Problem Based Learning meetings with discussion of the results)				■				
	Time to implement the changes					■			
Stage 4	Re-Audit (Data collection, analysis and reporting)						■		
	Writing final report							■	
	Public presentation of Audit final report								■

Fig. 2. Example of activity planning from a Clinical Audit - Gantt chart can be useful to summarize the audit plan

Facilitating factors	Barriers
Simplicity of design and ease of data collection (i.e. computerized medical records)	Lack of definition of the objectives Lack of details of the method
Strong leadership and management	Discontinuity in the organisational structure
Dedicated staff time and organisational facilities Good planning	Lack of management resources (time, suitable information systems, experience in planning of data collection and analysis, writing reports)
Final monitoring results	Lack of facilitating support (strategic and operational)
Positive climate (respect and trust between all actors)	Negative climate (difficult relationship)

Table 10. Facilitating factors and barriers to realize an audit in PC (modified from Potter et al, 2010).

3.5 Stage 4 of the Audit cycle: Sustaining improvements, re-audit

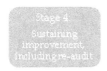

Did we improve?
Have we made things better?

After an agreed upon period of implementing changes, the data collection should be repeated (re-audit) (UBHT, 2005; Potter et al, 2010). A complete audit cycle ideally involves two data collections and a comparison of one with the other, following the implementation of change after the first data collection, in order to determine whether the desired improvements have been achieved *(Have we made things better?)*. Healthcare organisations are expected to provide assurance that new evidence-based healthcare interventions are being implemented, and that poor performance or substandard quality is being addressed and corrected. The second data collection may provide evidence that the changes implemented have had the desired effect and have led to improvements in quality *(Did we improve?)*. The same strategies for identifying the sample, methods and data analysis should be used to ensure comparability. The timing of the further phases of data collection is important, so that the second data collection provides valid and reliable data to be compared with those collected in the first data collection.

Collecting data for a second time, after changes have been introduced and have had time to bring about effect (figure 2), is central to both assessing and maintaining the improvements made during clinical audit. A re-audit should include all criteria where the original analysis demonstrated that acceptable levels of performance were not met and changes in practice were implemented. In table 11 the simple final report of the Clinical Audit, reported in figure 2, is shown as an example. Even if the Clinical Audit was successfully completed, many values did not improve enough to reach the ALP (Acceptable Level of Performance).

Recommendations (from GOLD guidelines, 2003)	Indicators	ALP*	First round Data		Re-AUDIT Data (after 6 months)	
			GPs pat (n. 174)	Hosp pat (n. 229)	GPs pat (n. 239)	Hosp pat (n. 207)
Brief tobacco dependence counseling is effective and every tobacco user should be offered at least this treatment at every visit to a health care provider. (Level of Evidence A)	% of COPD patients with tobacco history registered (last 2 ys)	≥70%	97 %	88 %	98%	93 %
	% of COPD patients with tobacco dependence counseling registered	≥50%	100 %	52%	100 %	74%
For the diagnosis and assessment of COPD, spirometry is the gold standard as it is the most reproducible, standardized, and objective way of measuring airflow limitation. FEV1/FVC < 70% and a post-bronchodilator FEV1 < 80% expected, confirms the presence of airflow limitation that is not fully reversible. (Level of Evidence A)	% of COPD patients with a registered spirometry (last 2 ys)	≥50%	54%	80%	70%	85%
	% of COPD patients with registered FVC and FEV1 (to define severity stage)	≥70%	11%	85%	25%	88%
Bronchodilator medications are central to the symptomatic management of COPD. They are given on an as-needed basis or on a regular basis to prevent or reduce symptoms. (Level of Evidence A)	% of COPD patients with at least one prescription (last year) of short acting bronchodilators in any stage of disease	≥90%	26%	43%	30%	47%
The addition of regular treatment with inhaled glucocorticosteroids (ICS) to bronchodilator treatment is appropriate for symptomatic COPD patients with an FEV1 <50% predicted (Stage III: Severe COPD and Stage IV: Very Severe COPD) and repeated exacerbations. (Level of Evidence A)	% of COPD patients with at least one prescription of ICS (last year) for stages III and IV and repeated exacerbations	≥70%	85%	90%	84%	91%
	% of COPD patients with at least one prescription of ICS (last year) for Stages I and II	≤20%	80%	80%	50%	65%

*ALP: Acceptable Level of Performance Blue value: ALP satisfied Red value: ALP not satisfied
GPs pat: patients from General Practitioners' databases - Hosp pat: patients from Pulmonary Clinic databases

Table 11. Final Report for the Clinical Audit cited in figure 2 – Comparison of data obtained before and after

Where further measurement is not deemed necessary, documented reasons are recommended to justify why this has not taken place. At this stage there may be justification for adjusting the desired performance levels in the light of the results obtained. If the expected results are not achieved, further cycles may be required. (Burgess, 2011).

The description of the conclusions is an essential part of the audit process, but one that is often omitted. Conclusions should be drawn as a team activity involving the whole audit team and other practice staff affected by the changes achieved in the audit process (Simon, 2008). The dissemination of audit results (both through management and governance systems and clinical channels) is an essential step to share methodology and solutions adopted to overcome barriers and involve participants and/or stakeholders (Potter et al, 2010).

Ongoing monitoring arrangements should be agreed upon and set in place following completion of the audit, in order to ensure that performance is maintained over time and in order to identify any reduction in quality. These may involve further routine 'snapshot' audits and/or make use of other feedback mechanisms that could indicate performance issues.

Improvements should be maintained and reinforced over time by ensuring that practical and user-friendly processes are built into systems. A culture that embraces change and encourages feedback will assist with the smooth transition from old to new ways of working (Burgess, 2011).

4. Significant Event Audit

Significant Event Audit (SEA) is a particular type of Audit, very suitable for Primary Care. SEA is a recognized methodology, peer review, used to analyze important events in a practice. SEA implies seven stages (Table 12). Discussion of specific events can identify learning objectives and provoke emotions that can be harnessed to achieve change. For it to be effective, it must be practiced in a culture that avoids blame and involves all disciplines (Simon, 2008).

5. Audit and training (Continuing Medical Education)

A clinical audit is a planned education activity designed to help general practitioners (GPs) to systematically review aspects of their own clinical performance in practice (RACGP, 2007). In 1976 Paul Sanazaro stated that the clinical audit and continuing medical education (CME) are the mainstays of quality assurance in health organisations. The quality assurance increasingly represents a near-guarantee of appropriate treatment and fewest possible complications for every patient. Maintenance of the public trust rests on a firm commitment of the medical staff and board to this principle, implemented through an organized program of quality assurance. Under these conditions, medical clinical audit and continuing medical education can effectively improve care by improving physician performance.

However, 20 years later the issue of mandatory continuing medical education (CME) is debated (Donen, 1998). Whilst ongoing educational development is an important value for a professional, and there is an ethical obligation to keep up-to-date, there is no evidence that current approaches to CME, mandatory or voluntary, may produce sustainable changes in

Stage	Actions to do	Some more informations...
1	Awareness and prioritisation of a significant event	Staff should be confident in their ability to identify and prioritise a significant event when it happens.
2	Information gathering	Collecting and collating as much factual information on the event as possible from personal testimonies, written records and other healthcare documentation.
3	The facilitated team-based meeting	The team should appoint a facilitator who will structure the meeting, maintain basic ground rules and help with the analysis of each event. The team should meet regularly to discuss, investigate and analyse events. An effective SEA should involve detailed discussion of each event, demonstration of insightful analysis, the identification of learning needs and agreement on any action to be taken.
4	Analysis of a significant event	The analysis of a significant event can be guided by answering four questions: 1. What happened? 2. Why did it happen? 3. What has been learned? 4. What has been changed or actioned?
5	Agreement, implementation and change monitoring	Any agreed action should be implemented by staff designated to co-ordinate and monitor change in the same way the practice would act on the results of 'traditional' audits.
6	Write it up	It is important to keep a comprehensive, anonymised, written record of every SEA, as external organisations will require evidence that the SEA was undertaken to a satisfactory standard. The SEA report is a written record of how effectively the significant event was analysed.
7	Report, share and review	Reporting when things go wrong is essential in general practice. The practice should formally report those events where patient safety has, or could have, been compromised.

Table 12. The seven stages of Significant Event Audit (adapted from Bowie & Pringle, 2008)

physician practices or application of current knowledge. Viceversa, mandating self-audit of the effect of individual learning on physician's practices and evaluation by the licensing authority are effective ways of ensuring the public are protected.

Today, junior doctors can find that audit is helpful to acquire an understanding of the healthcare process (Benjamin, 2008).

- Junior doctors need to experience directly that clinical audit is a quality improvement process; they should have the opportunity to work through the improvement process as part of their clinical audit experiences (Dixon, 2010). Carrying out clinical audits is one way by which an individual doctor can demonstrate initiative, interest, and commitment to progress in his or her career.

Junior doctors should seek to participate in all phases of the audit cycle. Thus they can enhance their prospects of audit data being used not only locally but also disseminated more widely. (Potter, 2010).

There are at least two reasons why a junior doctor at any level of training should be motivated to carry out clinical audits and therefore provide evidence of:

- meeting training requirements at the current level of training;
- showing why he or she is interested in and committed to the next step in their career (Dixon, 2010).

Learning and education of doctors, not only when training but also in post qualification and as part of continued professional development are critical components to ensure high quality and improving care.

Such learning needs to include not only the clinical aspects of care, but also personal development such as clinical leadership, change management and effective function with the organisation. Clinical audit and associated change management techniques must be an increasingly important part of medical practice and medical training (Potter, 2010).

6. Clinical Audit and Ethics

Quality improvement activity is essential among professionals and healthcare organisations and has widely brought about benefits for patients (Casarett et al, 2002; Dixon, 2009). This activity is strictly connected with Ethics, which is "the inquiry into certain situations and into the language employed to describe them; the kind of situations referred to are those that have led or may lead to harms or benefits to others". (Beauchamp & Childress, 1994).

Fundamental medical ethics assert (Childress, 1989; Eriksson et al, 2007; Tapp et al, 2010) that there are some principles to which doctors should abide:

- **Autonomy**: any person having the ability to make decisions should be treated with respect for that ability;
- **Utility:** benefit should be maximised and damage minimised;
- **Justice:** no person should be discriminated against, everyone should have equal access to equal treatment, and there should be solidarity with the less fortunate.

These basic medical principles should be used as a basis for judging the ethics of any system of quality improvement, including clinical audit.

On this basis, healthcare professionals, working in primary care settings, should actively participate in clinical audits and quality improvement projects for the same reasons as any other healthcare practitioners. Many primary care organisations are small, with a less formal accountability structure than the one existing in larger healthcare. It is less clear what method of ethics oversight of clinical audits and quality improvement activities might work best in these care settings (Burgess, 2011; Tapp et al, 2010).

Whereas widely accepted ethical standards exist for other activities in the clinical arena, the arrangements ensuring that clinical audit and quality improvement activities conform to appropriate ethical standards are fragmented, lack clarity and have not been clearly or thoroughly articulated (Deming, 1986; Dixon, 2009; Fox & Tulsky, 2005; Gerrish & Mawson, 2005; Langley et al, 2009).

The starting point in any consideration of ethics is that an audit project should benefit patients and not harm them. When properly conducted, clinical audits and other quality improvement activities can be seen as an ethical imperative in healthcare, something from which both professionals and patients benefit and with which they both should cooperate (Burgess, 2011; Jennings et al, 2007).

When trying to ameliorate practice through audit, a professional must be both sensitive to ethical responsibility and managing responsibility in order to satisfy the rights and interests of patients (Dixon, 2009; Jennings et al, 2007).

Ethics of clinical audit has been a neglected area up to now (Cave & Nichols, 2007; Dixon, 2009; Dubler et al, 2007; Lo & Groman, 2003), yet audit or the analysis of previously collected data may happen to be unethical (BMJ, 2012).

Some key principles can be used to identify a clinical audit or quality improvement activity that should have an ethical review at the proposal stage. They include the following:

-   **Each patient's right to self-determination is respected** (Burgess, 2011; Casarett et al, 2002; Diamond et al, 2004; Dubler et al 2007; Fox &Tulsky, 2005; Layer, 2003;)
-   **There is a benefit to existing or future patients or others that outweighs the potential burdens or risks** (Burgess, 2011; Cretin et al, 2000; Casarett et al, 2002; Diamond et al, 2004; Fox & Tulsky, 2005; Jennings et al, 2007; Layer, 2003; Wade, 2005)
-   **Each patient's privacy and confidentiality are preserved** (Burgess, 2011; Casarett et al, 2002; Diamond et al, 2004; Fox & Tulsky, 2005; Layer, 2003;)
-   **The activity is fairly distributed across patient groups** (Burgess, 2011; Casarett et al, 2002; Fox &Tulsky, 2005; Layer, 2003).

Ethical oversight of clinical audit and quality improvement on the part of healthcare organisations ensures that these activities protect patients and their rights, and contributes to improve quality and safety of patient care.

7. Conclusions

Clinical Audit definitely is a very important method to practice ethics in the Primary Care setting. Its aim is to lead professionals to accomplish quality of care both for patients and for public health services, using the most appropriate, safe and cost-effective instruments.

Clinical Audit is also an instrument for "health's democracy", as it allows comparisons between health services and can therefore lead to the equalization of health performances.

Clinical Audit in PC should be part of the usual way to work, where professionals share and compare their daily activity with evidence-based standards adapted to fit their settings. However, deep changes in the organisation of work are needed in order to introduce the Clinical Audit method in Primary Care steadily: clinical practice in PC is a hard, complex activity, that can be rarely assessed through a linear cause-effect approach. Too many ungovernable and unpredictable events occur between a physician's decision and a clinical outcome (i.e. understanding of information, patient's compliance, drugs tolerability, presence or absence of facilities in the local healthcare system, the domestic environment, etc.). Other constraining factors are the very habits, attitudes and motivations of the professionals themselves. Professionals and Health Service must share clinical data and information, the electronic standard of which is still unusual and therefore difficult to use. A virtuous process of improvement of professional conditions is fundamental, removing barriers to renovation and implementing really effective actions for the patients' sake.

Last but not least, Clinical Audit is a strong instrument for continuing medical education, as it requires the professionals to review their past experiences and knowledge, and therefore to behave in order to minimize the gap between best practice and current praxis.

8. References

Anderson DG. *ABC of audit*, Cleveland Vocational Training Scheme; accessed on February 2012:
http://www.gp-training.net/training/tutorials/management/audit/audabc.htm

Ashford J, Eccles M, Bond S, Hall LA, Bond J. (1999) Improving health care through professional behaviour change: introducing a framework for identifying behaviour change strategies. *British Journal of Clinical Governance;* 4(1): 14–23.

Baker R, Camosso-Stefinovic J, Gillies C, Shaw EJ, Cheater F, Flottorp S, Robertson N. (2010) Tailored interventions to overcome identified barriers to change: effects on professional practice and health care outcomes. *Cochrane Database Syst Rev;* (3):CD005470.

Baker R. & Fraser RC. (1995) Development of audit criteria: linking guidelines and assessment of quality. *BMJ,* 31: 370-3.

Beauchamp TL, & Childress JF. (1994) Principles of Biomedical Ethics. 4th ed. Oxford University Press.

Benjamin A. (2008) Audit: how to do it in practice. *BMJ;* 336:1241-5

Bhopal RS, Thomson R. (1991) A form to help learn and teach about assessing medical audit papers. *BMJ;* 303(6816):1520-2.

Black, N. (1992) The relationship between evaluative research and audit. *Journal of Public Health Medicine;* 14: 361–366.

BMJ anonymous. (2012) Ethics approval of research; accessed on February 2012: http://www.bmj.com/about-bmj/resources-authors/forms-policies-and-checklists/ethics- approval-research

Bowie P, Pringle M. (2008) Significant Event Audit, Guidance for Primary Care Teams, National Reporting and Learning Service, NHS; accessed on February 2012: http://www.rcgp.org.uk/pdf/CIRC_Significant_Event_Audit.pdf

Brain J, Schofield J, Gerrish K, Mawson S, Mabbott I, Patel D and Gerrish P. (2009) A Guide for Clinical Audit, Research and Service Review — An educational toolkit designed to help staff differentiate between clinical audit, research and service review activities; accessed on February 2012: http://www.hqip.org.uk/assets/Downloads/Audit-Research-Service-Evaluation.pdf

Brown P, Brunnhuber K, Chalkidou K, Chalmers I, Clarke M, Fenton M, Forbes C, Glanville J, Hicks NJ, Moody J, Twaddle S, Timimi H, Young P. (2006) How to formulate research recommendations. *BMJ*; 333: 804-6.

Burgess R. (2011) New Principles of Best Practice in Clinical Audit. Published by Radcliffe Publishing, Oxford, 2nd edition, ISBN- 13 :978-1-84619-221-0

Cabana MD, Rand CS, Powe NR, Wu AW, Wilson MH, Abbound PC, Rubin HR. (1999) Why don't physicians follow clinical practice guidelines? A framework for improvement. *JAMA*; 282(15): 458–65.

Campbell SM, Braspenning J, Hutchinson A, Marshall M. (2002), Research methods used in developing and applying quality indicators in primary care *Qual Saf Health Care*; 11:358-64.

Casarett D, Fox E, Tulsky JA. (2002) Recommendations for the Ethical Conduct of Quality Improvement; accessed on February 2012: http://www.ethics.va.gov/docs/necrpts/ NEC_Report_20020501_Ethical_Conduct_of_Quality_Improvement.pdf

Cave E, & Nichols C. (2007) Clinical audit and reform of the UK research ethics review system. *Theor Med Bioeth*; 28:181–203.

CCHSA (Canadian Council on Health Services Accreditation) (1996) A guide to the development and use of performance indicators. Published by *The Council* in Ottawa: *ID Numbers Open Library* OL21074209M

Chaillet N, Dube E, Dugas M, Audibert F, Tourigny C, Fraser W, Dumont A. (2006) Evidence-based strategies for implementing guidelines in obstetrics. *Obstetrics and Gynecology*; 108: 1234–45.

Childress JF. (1989) The normative principles of medical ethics. In Medical Ethics ed. Veatch RM, *Jones and Bartlett Publishers* Boston, pp 27-48.

Clark S. & Rowe F. (2002) Clinical Audit. *British Orthoptic Society:* accessed on February 2012: http://www.rcgp.org.uk/pdf/CIRC_British%20Orthoptic%20Society.pdf

Copeland, G. (2005) A practical handbook for clinical audit. Guidance published by the Clinical Governance Support Team; accessed on February 2012: www.cgsupport.nhs.uk/downloads/Practical_Clinical_Audit_Handbook_v1_1.pdf

Cretin S, Keeler EB, Lynn J Batalden, PB, Berwick DM, Bisognano M. (2000) Should patients in quality- improvement activities have the same protections as participants in research studies? *JAMA;* 284: 1786.

Crombie IK, Davies HTO, Abraham SCS, Florey CDV. (1993) The audit handbook-improving health care through clinical audit. 1st ed. *John Wiley & Sons* Chichester, ISBN:0-471-937665

Deming WE. (1986) Out of the Crisis: Quality, Productivity and Competitive Position. *Cambridge University Press*; ISBN   0911379010, 9780911379013.

Diamond LH, Kliger AS, Goldman RS,. Palevsky PM. (2004) Quality improvement projects: how do we protect patients' rights? *American Journal of Medical Quality*; 19: 25–7.

Dixon N, (2009) Review of Ethics Issues related to Clinical Audit and Quality Improvement Activities. *The Healthcare Quality Improvement Partnership (HQIP):* accessed on February 2012: http://www.hqip.org.uk/assets/Downloads/Ethics-and-Clinical-Audit-and-Quality-Improvement-Literature-Review.pdf

Dixon N, (2010) Guide to Involving Junior Doctors in Clinical Audit. *HQIP, Healthcare Quality Improvement Partnership;* accessed on February 2012: http://www.hqip.org.uk /assets/5-HQIP-CA-PD-026-Guide-to-Involving-Junior-Doctors-in-Clinical-Audit-19-April-2010.pdf

Donabedian A. (1966) Evaluating the quality of medical care. *Milbank Mem Fund Q;* 44 (3 suppl):166-206

Donen, N. (1998) No to mandatory continuing medical education, yes to mandatory practice auditing and professional educational development. *CMAJ;* 158, Issue 8: 1044

Dubler N, Blustein J, Bhalla R, Bernard D. (2007) Information participation: an alternative ethical process for including patients in quality-improvement projects. In: Jennings B, Baily MA, Bottrell M, Lynn J, editors. Health Care Quality Improvement: Ethical and Regulatory Issues. Garrison NY: The Hastings Center; p. 69–87.

Eccles M, Miiman B. (2006) Welcome to Implementation Science. *Implementation Science* [serial online] vol.1(1):[3 pages]; accessed on February 2012: http://www.implementationscience.com/content/1/1/1

EPOC Author Resources (2002) Cochrane Effective Practice and Organisation of Care Group, Data Collection Checklist; accessed on February 2012: http://www.epoc.cochrane.org/en/handsearchers.html.

Eriksson T, Nilstun T, Edwards A. (2007) The ethics of risk communication in lifestyle interventions: consequences of patient centeredness. *Health Risk Soc;* 9:19-36.

Ferlie E, Shortell S. (2001) Improving the quality of health care in the United Kingdom and the United States: a framework for change. *Milbank Q;* 79: 281–315.

Fitzpatrick R. Boulton M. (1994) Qualitative methods for assessing healthcare. *Quality in Health Care* vol: 3 pag: 107-13.

Fox E, Tulsky JA. (2005) Recommendations for the ethical conduct of quality improvement. *J Clin Ethics;*16(1):61–71.

Garside R. (1998) Organisational context for quality: lessons from the field of organisational development and change management. *Qual Health Care;* 7: S8–S15.

Gerrish K, Mawson S. (2005) Research, audit, practice development and service evaluation: Implications for research and clinical governance. *Practice Development in Health Care;* 4(1):33–9.

GOLD (2003). Global Strategy for Diagnosis, Management, and Prevention of COPD. Workshop final report; accessed on February 2012: http://www.goldcopd.org/uploads/users/files/GOLDWkshp2003Clean.pdf

Grimshaw JM, Thomas RE, MacLennan G, Fraser C, Ramsay CR, Vale L, Whitty P, Eccles MP, Matowe L, Shirran L, Wensing M, Dijkstra R, Donaldson C. (2004) Effectiveness and efficiency of guideline dissemination and implementation strategies, *Health Technology Assessment Monograph Series* Vol: 8(6): 1-72.

Grol R., Grimshaw J. (2003) From best evidence to best practice: effective implementation of change in patients' care. *Lancet;* 362(Issue 9391): 1225-1230.

Grol R, Wensing M, Eccles M. (2005) Improving patient care: the implementation of change in clinical practice. Elsevier Editor, Pages: 304, ISBN: 9780750688192

Grol R. (1997) Beliefs and evidence in changing clinical practice. *BMJ*; 315:418–21.

HQIP (Healthcare Quality Improvement Partnership) (2009) Criteria and indicators of best practice in clinical audit; accessed on February 2012: http://www.hqip.org.uk/assets/Downloads/Criteria-and-indicators-of-best-practice-in-clinical-audit.pdf

Hermens R (2011) International Forum on Quality and Safety in Healthcare, Amsterdam 5-8 april 2011; accessed on February 2012:
http://video.internationalforum.bmj.com /events/amsterdam-2011/sessions?tracks =Clinical%20improvement%20and%20innovation

Hogg W, Dyke E. (2011) Improving measurement of primary care system performance. *Can Fam Physician;* 57: 758-760.

Jamtvedt G, Young JM, Kristoffersen DT, O'Brien MA, Oxman AD (2006). Audit and feedback: effects on professional practice and health care outcomes. *Cochrane Database of Systematic Reviews* Issue 2. Art. No.: CD000259. DOI: 10.1002/14651858.

JCAHO (Joint Commission on Accreditation of Healthcare Organisations) (1989) Characteristics of clinical indicators. *Qual Rev Bull;* 11: 330–339.

Jennings B, Baily M.A, Bottrell M, Lynn J. (2007) Health Care Quality Improvement Ethical and Regulatory Issues, Garrison, NY: *The Hastings Center:* accessed on February 2012:
http://www.thehastingscenter.org/uploadedFiles/Publications/Special_Reports/Health%20Care%20Quality%20Improvement.pdf

Langley GJ, Moen RD, Nolan KM, Nolan TW, Norman CL, Provost LP. (2009) The Improvement Guide. A Practical Approach to Enhancing Organisational Performance, Second Edition, Published by Jossey-Bass, ISBN: 978-0-470-19241-2

Layer T. (2003) Ethical conduct recommendations for quality improvement projects. *Journal for Healthcare Quality;* 25: 44–6.

Lo B & Groman M. (2003) Oversight of quality improvement. *Arch Intern Med;*163: 1481–6.

Lomas J. (1994) Teaching old (and not so old) dogs new tricks: effective ways to implement research findings. In: Dunn EV, Norton PG, Stewart M, et al, eds. Chapter 1. Disseminating research/changing practice, Sage Publication, University Michigan, ISBN: 0803957068, EAN: 978-0803957060

M.E.R.G: Multi-professional Evidence-based practice and Research Group, (2012) NHS; Research & Development, accessed on February 2012:
http://www.researchdirectorate.org.uk/merg/documents/Audit%20Info.pdf

Mancey-Jones M, Brugha RF. (1997) Using perinatal audit to promote change: a review. Health Policy Plan;12:183-92

National Clinical Audit Advisory Group (NCAAG), accessed on February 2012 : http://www.dh.gov.uk/en/Publicationsandstatistics/Publications/PublicationsPolicyAndGuidance/DH_103396

National Institute for Clinical Excellence (2002), "Principles for Best Practice in Clinical Audit, Published by: *Radcliffe Medical Press*, ISBN: 1-85775-976-1: http://www.nice.org.uk/media/796/23/BestPracticeClinicalAudit.pdf

NICE (National Institute for Clinical Excellence) (2010) Management of chronic obstructive pulmonary disease in adults in primary and secondary care - Clinical guidelines, CG101 (This guideline partially updates and replaces NICE clinical guideline 12); accessed on February 2012: http://guidance.nice.org.uk/CG101

NHS Wirral (2012) Clinical Audit Team; accessed on February 2012: http://www.wirral.nhs.uk/aboutnhswirral/directorates/corporateaffairs/governanceteam/clinicalaudit.html

Pope C, Ziebland S, Mays N. (2000) Qualitative research in healthcare. Analysing qualitative data. *BMJ*; 320: 114-16.

Potter J, Fuller C, Ferris M. (2010) Local clinical audit: handbook for physicians. Healthcare Quality Improvement Partnership. Royal College of Physicians; August 2010; accessed on February 2012: http://www.hqip.org.uk

Powell J, Lovelock R, Bray I et al. (1994) Involving users in assessing service quality: benefits of using a qualitative approach. *Quality in Health Care*; 3: 199-202.

RACGP (Royal Australian College of General Practitioners) (2007) QA&CPD Program handbook for general practitioners: 2008–2010 triennium. Melbourne: The RACGP. http://www.racgp.org.au/Content/NavigationMenu/educationandtraining/TheGeneralPracticeMentalHealthStandardsCollaboration/AccreditationofmentalhealthtrainingforindividualGPs/GPMHSCGuidelines_ClinicalAudits.pdf

Robertson N, Baker R, Hearnshaw H. (1996) Changing the clinical behaviour of doctors - a psychological framework. *Quality in Health Care*; 5:51–4.

QOF (2012) - Quality and Outcomes Framework 2010/11; accessed on February 2012: http://www.ic.nhs.uk/qof

Scally G. & Donaldson L. J. (1998) Clinical governance and the drive for quality improvement in the new NHS in England. *BMJ*; 317(7150): 61-65.

Schofield J. & Jenkins J. (2009) How to Implement Local Changes from National Clinical Audit —A Guide for Audit Professionals in Healthcare Organisations; accessed on February 2012: http://www.hqip.org.uk/assets/Downloads/Implementing-Local-Change-from-National-Audit.pdf

Simon C. (2008) Audit in primary care. *InnovAiT*, Vol. 1, No. 4, pp. 281–287, 2008

Smith R. (1992) Audit & Research, *BMJ*; 305(6859):905-6

Starey N. (2001) 'What is clinical governance?' Evidence-based medicine, Hayward Medical Communications: http://www.medicine.ox.ac.uk/bandolier/painres/download/whatis/WhatisClinGov.pdf

Tapp L, Edwards A, Elwyn G, Holm S, Eriksson T. (2010) Quality improvement in general practice: enabling general practitioners to judge ethical dilemmas, *Journal of Medical Ethics*; 36: 184–8.

UBHT Clinical Audit Central Office (2005): How to do clinical audit - a brief guide.

UHBristol, NHS Foundation Trust, (2009), Clinical Audit Team:

http://www.uhbristol.nhs.uk/for-clinicians/clinicalaudit/how-to-guides/

Wade DT. (2005) Ethics, audit, and research: all shades of grey. *BMJ*; 330: 468–71.

Wienand U. (2009), Audit clinico: che cosa è e che cosa non è: l'uso inappropriato del termine depaupera il metodo. *QA*; 19(2): 82-90

Wollersheim H, Hermens R,. Hulscher M, Braspenning J, Ouwens M, Schouten J, Marres H, Dijkstra R, Grol R. (2007) Clinical indicators: development and applications. *Neth J Med*; 65(1):15-22.

Zwanenberg V & Harrison J. (2004) Clinical Governance in Primary Care. 2nd edition. Radcliffe Medical Press - ISBN 10: 1857758617.

8

Traditional Medicine and Complementary/Alternative Medicine in Primary Health Care: The Brazilian Experience

Caroline da Rosa

Fundação de Atendimento Sócio-Educativo do Rio Grande do Sul (FASE/RS)
Brazil

1. Introduction

Science has contributed a lot to longevity, as the discoveries of antibiotics and vaccines against diseases, for example, have been controlled or even extinct. But even with the hegemony of the biomedical model focused on allopathic medicine, the use of herbal and other therapeutic practices for the treatment of diseases has never been dropped. In an attempt to unite science and popular wisdom, medicine has been using more and more both practices to improve the quality of life.

Public health issues have always been a motive for reflection as they directly affect the quality of life of a nation. Making a socioeconomic, cultural and epidemiological analysis we realize that the changes in the modern world through the beginning of this century led to a social inequality and exclusion because of ineffective social policies and low public investment. Luz (2005) described the phenomenon of "health crisis" as an expression of an actual health crisis that generates levels of malnutrition, progressive increase in chronic degenerative diseases, new epidemics and diseases related to the collective malaise, such as anxiety, depression and panic. These diseases affect millions of individuals of the populations of almost every country in major cities, causing a situation of permanent suffering of the citizens and loss of many millions of dollars annually for the economies of these countries, in terms of days out of work and victims crowding the service of primary health care.

The scenario described has a direct impact on modern medicine. "Health crisis" paved the way for the institutionalization of other forms of treatment in public health service: Traditional Medicine and Complementary/ Alternative Medicine (TM/CAM) such as Homeopathy, Traditional Chinese Medicine and Herbal Medicine. These therapies have specific features in their practices, among these features is the attention and listening to patients and individualized therapy. Paradigmatic features of these medical rationalities, which put the patient in the center of medical activity, thus rescuing the art of healing (Araújo, 2008; Ferreira & Luz, 2007).

According to the World Health Organization (WHO), in 2011, between 70%, and 95% of citizens in a majority of developing countries, especially those in Asia, Africa, Latin America and the Middle East, were using traditional medicine, including herbal medicines, for the management of health and as primary health care to address their health-care needs and concerns. In addition, in some industrialized nations the use of traditional medication is equally significant. For instance: Canada, France, Germany and Italy, report that between 70% and 90% of their populations have used traditional medicines under the titles "complementary", "alternative", or "nonconventional" (WHO, 2011). Since the late 70's, in various statements and resolutions, the WHO has expressed its commitment to encourage the formulation and implementation of public policies for integrated and rational use of Traditional Medicine and Complementary/Alternative Medicine in national health care as well as the development of studies for better scientific knowledge of its safety and efficacy. The document "WHO Strategy on Traditional Medicine 2002 - 2005" (WHO, 2002a) reaffirms the development of these principles.

Traditional Medicine and Complementary/Alternative Medicine introduced into the primary health care in the health system involves approaches that seek to encourage natural mechanisms of prevention and treatment of health disorders through safe and effective technologies. Furthermore, this approach is based on the emphasis in developing a therapeutic relationship and the integration of humans with the environment and society. Other points shared by the various approaches within this field are the broader view of the health-disease process and overall promotion of human care, especially self-care.

Brazil is the largest country in South America. It is the world's fifth largest country, both by geographical area and by population with over 190 million people (Brasil, 2011). In this country the legitimization and institutionalization of these approaches to health care were initiated in the 80's, especially after the creation of the Unified Health System (SUS) (Brasil, 1990). The SUS was created as part of the 1988 Federal Constitution to ensure that all Brazilians have universal, integral and equal access to public health care. It constitutes of a health system based on the undisputed premise of the Declaration of Alma-Ata, fruit of the "International Conference on Primary Health Care" in 1978 (WHO/UNICEF, 1978). For the Brazilian law *"health is everyone's right and duty of the state, guaranteed through social and economic policies aiming at reducing the risk of any illness and other disorders and providing universal and equalitarian access to actions and services for its promotion, protection, and recovery"*.

The SUS is characterized by the decentralization of actions and popular participation, which allowed states and cities to gain more autonomy in setting their policies and actions in health, contributing for the growth of pioneering experiments. This scenario was favorable to an innovative health policy, as the case of the National Policy of Integrative and Complementary Practices (PNPIC) in 2006 (Brasil, 2006a; Brazil 2008).

2. National Policy of Integrative and Complementary Practices (PNPIC) in the Unified Health System (SUS), Brazil

The PNPIC was published in the Brazilian Official Gazette in May 2006. This policy caters mainly the need to understand, support, incorporate, and implement experiences with Integrative Practices that had already been developed in primary health care in many cities and states.

Among these health practices, we can highlight those in the Traditional Chinese Medicine, Acupuncture, Homeopathy, Herbal Medicine, Anthroposophical Medicine, and Hydrotherapy-Crenotherapy. These integrative practices are described below according to the definitions found in the PNPIC (Brasil, 2006a; Brazil, 2008).

2.1 Traditional Chinese Medicine

The Traditional Chinese Medicine is characterized by an essential medical system, originated thousands of years ago in China. It uses language that portrays symbolically the laws of the nature and that it values the harmonic interrelation among the parts seeking integrality. Having Yin-Yang as the fundamental basis, the division of the world in two forces of fundamental principles, interpreting all phenomena in complementary opposites.

The objective of this knowledge is to obtain means of balancing such duality. It also includes the theory of the five movements that attributes all things and phenomena in nature as well as in the body, one of the five energies (wood, fire, earth, metal, and water). The Traditional Chinese Medicine uses elements of anamnesis, palpation of the pulse, and the observation of the face and of the language in its several treatment modalities.

Traditional Chinese Medicine includes acupuncture; corporal practices (lian gong, chi gong, tui-na, tai-chi-chuan); mental practices (meditation); diet orientation; and the use of medicinal plants (Traditional Chinese Phytotherapy), related to the prevention of injuries and diseases, health promotion and recovery.

All treatment modalities are important and are covered in the PNPIC, acupuncture will be deeply studied in this chapter.

2.1.1 Acupuncture

Acupuncture is a health intervention technology that approaches in an integral and dynamic way the health-disease process in the human being, and could be used alone or in an integrated way with other therapeutic resources. Original of the Traditional Chinese Medicine, acupuncture comprises a group of procedures which allows the necessary stimulus of specific anatomical places through the insertion of threadlike metallic needles for the promotion, maintenance and recovery of health, as well as for the prevention of injuries and diseases.

Archeological findings allow us to suppose that this knowledge source remounts from at least 3,000 years. The Chinese denomination zhen jiu, which means needle (zhen) and heat (jiu) was adapted in the reports brought by the Jesuits in the 17th century, resulting in the word acupuncture (derived from the Latin words acus, needle and punctio, puncture). The therapeutic effect of the stimulation of neuroreactive areas or "acupuncture points" was first described and explained in a language of time, symbolic and analogical, consonant with the Chinese classic philosophy.

In the western societies, starting from the second half of the 20th century, acupuncture was assimilated by the contemporary medicine, and thanks to the scientific researches undertaken at several countries both eastern and western, their therapeutic effects were recognized and they have been explained gradually in scientific works published in respected scientific magazines (Aune et al., 1998; Ballegaard et al., 1990; Bullock et al., 1989; David et al., 1998; Diehl, 1999; Dundee et al., 1987; Jobst et al., 1986; Joshi, 1992; Lao et al., 1995; Lee et al., 1992; Petrie & Hazleman, 1986; Vincent, 1989; Vilholm et al., 1998; Washburn et al., 1993; Wong et al., 1999). It is now admitted that the stimulation of acupuncture points provokes the release, in the Central Nervous System, of neurotransmitters and other substances responsible for the responses of pain relieve promotion, restoration of organic functions and immunity modulation.

WHO recommends acupuncture to its Member States. In 2003 the WHO published a document entitled "Acupuncture: Review and analysis of reports on controlled clinical trials" in which presents the results of controlled clinical trials. In this paper it was analyzed the effectiveness of acupuncture compared with conventional treatment of 147 diseases, symptoms and health conditions (WHO, 2003).

In Brazil, acupuncture was introduced about 40 years ago. In 1988, through the Resolution no. 5/88 of the Planning and Coordination Interministerial Commission (Ciplan) (cited in Brasil, 2006a), acupuncture had their norms established for the service in the public health service. Several Health Professional Councils recognize acupuncture as a specialty in our country, and training courses are available in several states.

According to the diagnosis made by the Ministry of Health in 2004 (Brasil, 2006a; Brazil, 2008) found that acupuncture was present in 19 states, distributed in 107 municipalities and 17 capitals.

2.2 Homeopathy

Homoeopathy is a complex medical system bases on holistic and vital principle and in the use of the natural law of healing which was enunciated by Hippocrates in the 6th century b.C. It was developed by Samuel Hahnemann in the 18th century. After studies and reflections based on clinical observation and in experiments accomplished at the time, Hahnemann systematized the philosophical principles and doctrinaire of homeopathy in his works "Organon of the Art of Healing" and "Chronic Diseases". Since then, this medical thinking has experienced great expansion in different places of the world, and today it is firmly established at several countries of Europe, America and Asia.

In Brazil, homeopathy was introduced by Benoit Mure in 1840, and has become a new treatment option. In 1979, the Brazilian Homeopathic Medical Association was founded. In 1980, homeopathy was recognized as a medical specialty by the Federal Council of Medicine (Conselho Federal de Medicina, 1980). In the 1980s, some Brazilian states and municipalities started to offer homeopathic services as a medical specialty to the users of public health services, but as isolated initiatives and, sometimes discontinued because of the absence of a national policy. In 1988, with the Resolution no. 4/88, CIPLAN (cited in Brasil, 2006a), established rules for the service in Homeopathy in the public health services and, in 1999, the Ministry of Health places in the SUS template the medical consultation in homeopathy

With the establishment of SUS and the decentralization of the management, the homeopathy service increased. Such progress can be observed in the number of homeopathy consultations that, since its placement as a procedure in the SUS template, is showing an annual growth around 10%. In 2003, the SUS information system and the diagnosis data done by the Ministry of Health in 2004 showed that homeopathy is present in the public health network in 20 states, 16 capitals, 158 municipalities, counting with 457 homeopathy medical professionals registered.

Homeopathy is present in at least 10 public universities, in teaching, research or attention activities, and counts with courses for training Homeopathy specialists in 12 states. It also counts with training of Homeopathy Doctors approved by the National Commission of Medical Residence. Despite an increase of the services offered, the pharmaceutical attention in homeopathy does not follow this tendency. According to a survey done in 2000 by Brazilian Homeopathic Medical Association (Brasil, 2006a; Brazil, 2008), only 30% of the homeopathy services of the SUS network supplied homeopathic medicines. In 2003, in The report of the 1st National Conference on Medicines and Pharmaceutical Care, held in 2003 (Brasil, 2005) recommends "Establish mechanisms that facilitate the provision of homeopathic medicines to SUS users through the deployment of homeopathic pharmacies in public " and "ensure that private homeopathic pharmacies are complementary to the public health service providing users with full access to homeopathic medicines" .

The survey data done by the Ministry of Health in 2004, revealed that only 9.6% of the municipalities which informed having homeopathy services had Public Manipulation Pharmacies.

2.3 Medicinal plants and phytotherapy

Phytotherapy is a "therapeutic process characterized by the use of medicinal plants in their different pharmaceutical forms, without the use of isolated active substances, although of vegetable origin". The use of medicinal plants in the art of healing is an ancient form of treatment, related to the origins of the medicine and based in the accumulation of information by successive generations. Along the centuries, products of vegetable origins constituted the basis for treatment of different diseases.

Since the Declaration of Alma-Ata in 1978, WHO has been stating its position regarding the need of valuing the use of medicinal plants in the sanitary scope, knowing that 80% of the world population use those plants on preparations in what refers to the primary health attention. Besides that, it stands out the participation of developing countries in such process, since they have 67% of the world's vegetable species (WHO/UNICEF, 1978).

Brazil possesses great potential for the development of such therapeutics, as the country with the largest vegetable diversity in the world, wide social diversity, the use of medicinal plants linked to the traditional knowledge and technology to scientifically validate such knowledge. In fact, some medicinal plants and herbal medicines were evaluated in clinical trials, scientifically proven supported by evidence-based medicine (Blumenthal et al., 1998; WHO, 1999, 2002b).

In Brazil, the popular and institutional interest has been growing in the sense of strengthening phytotherapy in SUS. This theme and subsequent insertion of phytotherapy in the health service was the result of a long walk (Rosa et al., 2011). This subject was raised on several occasions, as in 1986, the 8th National Health Conference (Brasil, 1986), when it was recommended the introduction of traditional healing practices in public health care. Some initiatives that incorporate the use of available scientific and popular knowledge have shown promising results and visible growth, as the project "Living Pharmacies" (Matos, 1998), Federal University of Ceará (UFC), organized under the influence of the WHO recommendations on the use of medicinal plants in programs for primary health care.

Below the main documents and publications that guarantee phytotherapy in SUS:

- 1988. It was published the Ciplan resolution no 8/88 (cited in Brasil, 2006a),, which regulates the implementation of phytotherapy in the health services and creates procedures and routines related to its practice in the medical units;
- 1996. The Report of the 10th National Health Conference, held in 1996 (Brasil, 1998a), which states in: "to incorporate in SUS, through the entire country, the practices of health such as phytotherapy, acupuncture and homeopathy, contemplating the alternative therapies and popular practices" and in another item: "the Ministry of Health should stimulate phytotherapy use in the public pharmaceutical assistance and elaborate norms for its use, thoroughly discussed with health professionals and specialists, in cities where larger popular participation is a reality and with more engaged managers to the issue of citizenship and popular movements".
- 1998. The Administrative Rule no. 3916/98 (Brasil, 1998b), which approved the National Drugs Policy, which establishes in the scope of its guidelines for scientific and technological development: "… it should be continued and expanded the support to research that seek the use of the therapeutic potential of our flora and national fauna, emphasizing the certification of their medicinal potential".
- 2003. The report of the 1st National Conference on Medicines and Pharmaceutical Care, held in 2003 (Brasil, 2005) which among its recommendations states:
  - Provide a review of the Brazilian Pharmacopoeia, including and extending it in relation to herbal products, taking into account the regional character;
  - Support and encourage funding for research and development of the practice of organic farming of medicinal plants and deployment of services using herbal medicines in the public with the support of state and federal government;
  - Define and standardize herbal medicine services, organized by level of complexity of health care, with skilled human resources, incorporating traditional knowledge;
  - Develop in public universities, public research institutions and official laboratories, scientific research to the production of drugs, including studying and preserving the flora and fauna of Brazil, which meet local and regional needs;
  - Develop projects to encourage the production and rational use of herbal medicines.
- 2003. The report of the 12th National Health Conference held in 2003 (Brasil, 2003), which points out the need of "investing in research and technology development for the production of homeopathic medicines and medicines from the Brazilian flora, favoring the national production and the implementation of programs for the use of homeopathic medicines in the health services, in accordance with the recommendations of the 1st National Conference on Medicines and Pharmaceutical Care (Brasil, 2005)".
- 2004. The Resolution no 338/04 from the National Health Council (Brasil, 2004a) which approves the National Policy of Pharmaceutical Assistance, that contemplates in its strategic axes, the "definition and agreement of intersectorial actions which intends the use of the medicinal plants and herbal medicine in the process of health attention, respecting the traditional knowledge incorporated with scientific rationale, adopting policies of generation of work and income, with training and establishment of

procedures, involving the health professionals in the process of incorporation of this therapeutic option and based on the incentive to the national production, with the use of the existent biodiversity in the country".

* 2006. In June, the same month the National Policy of Integrative and Complementary Practices was published (Brasil, 2006a; Brazil, 2008), the National Policy of Medicinal Plants and Herbal Medicines was also published (Brasil, 2006b), prepared by the Interministerial Working Group formed by representatives of the Ministries of Health, National Integration, Development, Industry and Foreign Trade, Agricultural Development, Science and Technology, Environment, Agriculture, Livestock and Supply; Social Development and Fight Against Hunger, in addition to the National Agency of Sanitary Surveillance, Oswaldo Cruz Foundation (Fiocruz) and the Civil House. This policy includes guidelines that go beyond the spheres of the health care sector and covers the entire production chain of medicinal plants and herbal products. Through the actions arising out of this policy the government in partnership with the company seeks to ensure access to the Brazilian population safe and rational use of medicinal plants and herbal medicines, promoting the sustainable use of biodiversity, the development of the productive chain and national industry.

In a survey done by the Ministry of Health in 2004 (Brasil, 2006a; Brazil, 2008) it was verified that in all Brazilian municipalities phytotherapy is present in 116 municipalities, contemplating 22 states. There are state and municipal programs of phytotherapy, from those with therapeutic memento and specific regulation for the service, implemented more than 10 years ago, to those recently started or with intention for implementation.

2.4 Anthroposophical Medicine

Anthroposophical Medicine was introduced in Brazil approximately 60 years ago and consists of a complementary medical/therapeutic approach with a vitalistic orientation, with a care model organized in a cross-disciplinary manner seeking the integrality of health care. Anthroposophical doctors use the Anthroposophical Medicine knowledge and resources as tools to expand clinical treatment, and their practice was accredited by the Federal Medical Board's Opinion 21/93 of Nov. 23, 1993 (Conselho Federal de Medicina, 1993).

Resources supporting this medical approach include the use of homeopathic and herbal medicines and specific anthroposophical medicines. It provides for the activity of other health professionals integrated with the doctor's work, according to the specificities of each category.

Experiences in public health have offered contributions to the fields of people's education, art, culture, and social developments. There are a few experiences at the SUS, including the service of "non-allopathic practices" in Belo Horizonte, in which Anthroposophical Medicine was officially introduced into the municipal network, together with Homeopathy and Acupuncture (Brasil, 2008a). In 1996, the Municipal Department of Health of Belo Horizonte conducted the first specific competitive examination for admission of an anthroposophical doctor into the SUS. In November 2004, the service completed 10 years of existence, with an ever-increasing number of patients seen.

In the municipal public network in São João Del Rei, Minas Gerais, a multi-disciplinary Family Health team has developed for more than six years an innovative experience based on the use of external applications of herbal medicines and other approaches (Brasil, 2008b).

In addition, the outpatient facility of the Monte Azul Community Association in São Paulo has offered care based on this approach for 25 years, as an informal part of the local referral network, with a non-allopathic practice center (massage, art therapy, and external applications) (Associação Comunitária Monte Azul/SP, 2011). Since 2001, the Association has had a partnership with the Municipal Department of Health for the implementation of the Family Health Strategy in that municipality.

Due to its reduced presence at the SUS and based on initial positive evaluations on the insertion of the services, this Anthroposophical Medicine Policy proposes the implementation of Observatories, based on the consolidated experiences, to deepen knowledge on their practices and impact on health.

2.5 Social thermalism/crenotherapy

Thermalism constitutes the different ways of mineral water use and its application in health treatments. Crenotherapy consists of the prescription and use of mineral water with therapeutic purposes in a complementary way to other health treatments.

The use of mineral water in the treatment of health is a very ancient procedure, used from the time of the Greek Empire. It was described by Herodotus (450 B.C.), the author of the first scientific publication on thermalism.

In Brazil, crenotherapy was introduced with the Portuguese colonization, which brought to the country the habits of using mineral water for health treatment. For some decades it was considered a valuable and highly respected discipline present in medical schools such Federal University of Minas Gerais (UFMG) and Federal University of Rio de Janeiro (UFRJ). After the end of the Second World War, this field of study suffered considerable reduction of its scientific production and popularization with the changes in the field of medicine and of the social health production as a whole.

Starting from the decade of 1990s, the Thermal Medicine started to be dedicated to collective approaches, as much of prevention as of promotion and recovery of health, inserting in this context the concept of Health Tourism and Social Thermalism, whose main objective is the search and the maintenance of health.

European countries like Spain, France, Italy, Germany, Hungary, among others, adopt Social Thermalism since the beginning of the 20th century, as a way of presenting to senior people treatments in specialized thermal establishments, aiming to provide with the senior people the access to the use of the mineral water with medicinal properties, to health recovery as well as health maintenance.

Thermalism, had an active role in some municipal health services with thermal sources, as it is the case of Poços de Caldas in Minas Gerais.

The Administrative Rule from the National Health Council no 343 of October, 2004 (Brasil, 2004b) is an instrument of empowerment of the definition of government actions that involves the revaluation of mineral water springs, its therapeutic aspect, and the definitions of mechanisms of prevention, supervision, and control, besides the incentive for research in the area.

3. Brazilian experiences with Traditional Medicine and Complementary/Alternative Medicine in the Unified Health System (SUS)

3.1 Homeopathy used in fight against Dengue

Dengue is an example of a disease that may constitute a public health emergency of international concern with immense economic and social impact. It is transmitted by the *Aedes aegypti*, is the most rapidly spreading mosquite-borne viral disease in the world. Data released by the WHO (2009) show that, in the last 50 years, incidence has increased 30-fold with increasing geographic expansion to new countries and, in the present decade, from urban to rural settings. An estimated 50 million dengue infections occur annually and approximately 2,5 billion people live in dengue endemic countries. In Southern Cone countries (Brazil, Argentina, Chile, Paraguay e Uruguay) in the period from 2001 to 2007, 2, 798,601 of dengue cases were notified of which 6,733 were Dengue Hemorrhagic Fever with a total of 500 deaths. Some 98.5% of the cases were notified by Brazil which also reports the highest case fatality rate.

Symptoms of the sickness may initially be confused with a cold. There are two kinds of dengue, the classic, named Dengue Fever or just Dengue and the Dengue Hemorrhagic Fever. The Dengue Hemorrhagic Fever has all the clinical symptoms of classic one, which starts with a fever, splitting headache, pain in the eyes, severe muscle and joints pain, plus hemorrhagic symptoms that go from bleeding gums, nosebleeds, the appearance of marks on the skin, and some more serious cases, stomach bleedings (Centers for Disease Control and Prevention, 2011). People who think they have dengue should rest, drink plenty of fluids to prevent dehydration and consult a physician. For Dengue Hemorrhagic Fever, if a clinical diagnosis is made early, a health care provider can effectively treat Dengue Hemorrhagic Fever using fluid replacement therapy. Adequately management of Dengue Hemorrhagic Fever generally requires hospitalization.

There is not a vaccine yet or even specific medication for treatment of a dengue infection. Thus the only strategy to fight outbreaks of the disease is the control of the mosquito *Aedes aegypti* proliferation.

The experience of homeopathy to fight Dengue in Brazil was described by two researches, Marino (2008) in the city of São José do Rio Preto, state of São Paulo and Nunes (2008) in the city of Macaé, state of Rio de Janeiro. Both cities are located in the Southeast, the region with the largest population of the country.

Marino (2008), described the use of the homeopathic remedy *Eupatorium perfoliatum* in dilution 30cH in single doses to prevent Dengue fever. The study was conducted in the Cristo Rei area, the neighborhood with the highest incidence of Dengue in São José do Rio Preto in May 2001. The remedy was chosen by applying the principles of epidemic genus, considering the symptoms obtained in patients residing in the same neighborhood between March and April 2001 with confirmed diagnosis of Dengue. At the time, 4,850 residents lived in the neighborhood, 1,959 individuals (40.2%) took the homeopathic remedy. After the homeopathic intervention, Dengue incidence decreased by 81.5%, a highly significant decrease as compared with neighborhoods that did not receive homeopathic prophylaxis ($p < 0.0001$). Decrease in the number of cases in the neighborhoods considered between the first period - incidence of Dengue from January 1st to May 4th 2001- and the second period - reported cases from May 5th to December 31st 2001 - dramatically demonstrates the fall in incidence in Cristo Rei area. The author does not examine biases or factors that may have confounded this association.

Six years after this experience, in 2007, facing an aggravation of the epidemiological status of Dengue in São José do Rio Preto and neighboring counties, the Municipal Secretary of Health and Hygiene (SMSH) decided to implement the actions indicated in National Policy of Integrative and Complementary Practices for the national public health system. In this context, a homeopathic complex composed of *Eupatorium perfoliatum, Phosphorus* and *Crotalus horridus* - all in dilution 30cH, in a single dose of 2 drops p.o. was administered for Dengue prevention. It was hoped that such prophylaxis would attenuate the intensity of symptoms of Dengue and prevent hemorrhagic complications. From March 15th to 22nd 2007, 20,000 doses of homeopathic complex against Dengue were administered to the population of São José do Rio Preto, in accordance with the Health Secretary program aimed at including this resource in the ongoing fight to combat Dengue fever. The use of the homeopathic complex was restricted to this single week in March 2007 due to a disagreement between the State and Municipal Secretaries of Health giving rise to a serious institutional crisis widely reported by Brazilian media, creating feelings of doubt and confusion among the population. This situation also seriously impeded this research, limited to a small sample and inadequate controls (Marino, 2008).

Since the experiment conducted in the state of Rio de Janeiro, city of Macaé with complex homeopathic *Eupatorium perfoliatum, Phosphorus* and *Crotalus horridus* - all in dilution 30cH proposed by Marino (2008) could be completed without political and administrative problems. The remedy was prescribed in single doses, 2 drops p.o. for prevention purposes. In symptomatic cases suggesting dengue, the patient received at the public outpatient clinic a 5 ml vial of homeopathic remedy, to take 5 drops p.o. 3 times a day for one week. Educational materials were distributed among the population, explaining features of homeopathy: composition of remedies, expected effect, target population, side-effects, corresponding legislation, prevention regarding the mosquito and information on the disease and the fluxogram of treatment. Health workers were specifically trained; a "Routine for the assistance of patients suspected of dengue" included a protocol for the use of homeopathy. The estimated population of Macaé was 180,000 inhabitants. 156,000 doses of homeopathic remedy were freely distributed in April and May 2007 to asymptomatic patients and 129 doses to symptomatic patients treated in outpatient clinics. The incidence of the disease in the first three months of 2008 fell 93% by comparison to the corresponding period in 2007, whereas in the rest of the State of Rio de Janeiro there was an increase of 128%. While confounding factors were not controlled for, these results suggest that homeopathy may be an effective adjunct in Dengue outbreak prevention (Nunes, 2008).

Using these data, a Brazilian pharmaceutical company, registered homeopathic complex *Eupatorium perfoliatum, Phosphorus* and *Crotalus horridus* in dilution 30cH developed by Marino (2008) in National Health Surveillance Agency (ANVISA). Since December 2008, this product can be purchased at pharmacies and drugstores.

3.2 Alternative Medicine Hospital – Goiânia/Goiás

The city of Goiânia is the capital of the state of Goiás, located in the central region of the country. According to the census conducted by the Brazilian Institute of Geography and Statistics in 2010, Goiânia is the twelfth most populous city in Brazil with 1,302,001 inhabitants (Brasil, 2011). The Alternative Medicine Hospital (HMA) in the city of Goiânia has been running, maintained by the State Secretary of Health. Despite the name this institution as a hospital only has outpatient care.

The pioneer history Alternative Medicine Hospital began in August 1986, when an agreement was established between the Secretary of Health of the State of Goiás, Ministry of Health of Brazil and the Brazilian Institute of Science and Technology Maharishi (IBCTM). The first action taken by the new institution was the creation of the first course about Ayurvedic Phytotherapy, ancient therapeutic method of Indian origin, unheard in Brazil until then. In February 1987 an outpatient service and a small pharmaceutical laboratory were implemented, which served as internship for the doctors and pharmacist students. In April 1988 this service was transferred to a location where it still works today, and in September 1988 became a specialized hospital belonging to the chain of the Secretary of Health of the State of Goiás and received the current name: Alternative Medicine Hospital (Secretária da Saúde do Estado de Goiás, 2011a).

The care service that the HMA aims to achieve is harmonization of the individual. Understanding the patient holistically and investigating all possibilities for the total stabilization of the patient, this service seeks to promote and maintain health care in primary care. For this purpose appointments, group therapy, lectures and consultations with other health professionals such as pyshologists, nutritionists, nurses, speech therapists, physiotherapists and social works are offered.

The HMA has a garden, a unique experience in the public health in Brazil. In this case the local medicinal plant identification, growing and harvesting guided by specialized agronomists.

The number of consultations were reported in the HMA. In the year 2007 were 7,191 specialty consultations in herbal medicine, 10,109 consultations in the specialty of homeopathy, acupuncture consultations in 2,058 and 10,472 visits in other fields: psychology, nutrition, social work, nursing and physiotherapy. In 2010 were 5,963 specialty consultations in herbal medicine, 7,356 consultations in the specialty of homeopathy, in acupuncture consultations 1,777 and 13,135 visits in other fields: psychology, nutrition, social work, nursing and physiotherapy (Secretária da Saúde do Estado Góias, 2011b).

3.3 The corporal practice Lian Gong - Traditional Chinese Medicine in the city of Suzano/ São Paulo

The Lian Gong is a corporal practice established in the 70's by Dr. Zhuang Yuan Ming, a doctor of Traditional Chinese Medicine orthopedic surgeon who lives in Shanghai, China. The word "Lian" means train, but also to forge and "Gong" means work, experience, skill. That is, train and exercise a prolonged and persistent work that achieves a high level of skill (Lee, 2006).

This exercise technique was developed to prevent and treat pain in the body and restore its natural movement. The practice of Lian Gong is based on the same basic concepts of Traditional Chinese Medicine that underlie the Tui Na massage, acupuncture, Chinese herbal medicine and Qi Gong: Qi, Meridians and the Yin and Yang. Exercises are preventive and curative, whose practice sets in motion the "Chi" (vital energy) in particular the "Zhen Chi" or "Chi True" in the body, these terms found in the fundamentals of Traditional Chinese Medicine, which advocates the following: "When the Zhen Chi is fully inside the human body, the negatives can not invade".

According to Lee (2006) Lian Gong regularly practiced strengthens the health, strengthens and enhances the therapeutic effect, shortens the treatment time. For sedentary people, Lian Gong provides balancing motion and rest, preserving the functioning of the body and prevents disease. It operates in internal organ disorders and respiratory problems. It also helps in blood circulation, dissolve adhesions and inflammation of the tendons.

Thus, the Lian Gong is an exercise therapy for the treatment and prevention of diseases but also for longevity.

In the city of Suzano - located in the state of São Paulo with 262,568 inhabitants (Brasil, 2011) Lian Gong was implemented in an orderly fashion in 1999. Initially it aimed to promote care for the users of the municipal health monitoring programs of hypertension and diabetes (Brazil, 2008c). In October 2006, however, the Lian Gong became more visible when the city was the one selected by the Ministry of Health to invest in the experience of practice as a way of expanding health promotion activities in the municipality. The city acquired resources to be used specifically in the growth of this practice as an incentive for Surveillance and Prevention of Disease and Non-Communicable Diseases, with emphasis on corporal practices and physical activity.

Currently the city of Suzano estimates that more than 2,200 people across the city are adept at Lian Gong, mostly female. A survey of 150 practitioners of last year, pointed out interesting data on the Chinese corporal practice: most of the practioners are in the age range between 50 to 70 years. Most of these people are referred by the Family Health Strategy[1], to complement the treatment in controlling blood pressure - main complaint indicated by the survey (Brazil, 2008c).

Of these 150 people, 47% said that the number of doctors prescriptions were reduced after the adoption of the practice of Lian Gong, 83% of respondents admitted mood enhancement and 80% said there was improvement in feeding, sleep and expansion of social networking and family.

According to the Municipal Health Secretary, the Lian Gong is now a social achievement. There are 32 groups in activity in Suzano, eight monitors that rely on the work of Community Health Agents[2] and trained volunteers who are responsible for conducting classes. The average number of popular participation in each of these groups is 70 people.

---

[1] In Brazil, Family Health is understood as a strategy for reorienting the care model, operationalized through the implementation of multidisciplinary teams in health care. These teams are responsible for monitoring a number of families, located in a defined geographical area. The teams with the actions of health promotion, prevention, recovery, rehabilitation of most frequent diseases and disorders, and in maintaining the health of the community served.

[2] Team member of the Family Health Strategy. It is a resident of community served the position which has to be an essential link between the community and the health system.

The regular activities are carried out in the Basic Health Unit / Family Health (UBS / SF) and other community centers throughout the city.

3.4 Phytotherapy in the Basic Health Units – Vitória/Espírito Santo

The city of Vitória is the capital of the state of Espírito Santo, located in the southeast region with 325,453 inhabitants (Brasil, 2011). A survey conducted by the city of Vitória, in 1990, pointed out the 1,000 families interviewed, 95% had the habit of using herbs medicines and teas to treat some diseases, before seeking medical attention. Flu, colds, dyspepsia and worms were the most common diseases treated by the citizens who responded to interview (Brasil, 2008d).

Another survey was conducted with professionals from the municipal health care, where it was observed that the 44 doctors interviewed, 61.3% had an interest in prescribing herbal medicines to their patients. With these data, the Municipal Health Secretary introduced the Herbal Medicine Program in Vitória. The justification of program implementation was the integration of popular knowledge and medical practice, making it a therapeutic option, respecting pharmacological and clinical criteria.

However, the program only became institutionalized in 1996 and that same year, the city opened the Herbal Medicines Pharmacy. The pharmacy then went to work with several medicinal plants, offering users the primary care natural medicines of great acceptance and with less risk side. Since 1998, with the implementation of the Family Health Strategy in Vitória, the dispensing of these drugs has to be made in the Basic Health Units (UBS), by prescription. Subsequently, some herbal medicines selected were included in the Municipal Register of Essential Medicines (REMUME).

The Herbal Medicines Pharmacy was in operation in the city until 2004, when the city opted for the acquisition of manufactured drugs through purchase complying with certain criteria of public administration.

The Municipal Health Secretary provides healthcare professionals of Primary Care/Family Health with training courses in herbal medicine, available for physicians and community health agents. The course is divided into: a survey of the traditional use through home visits, identification of most often cited botanical species; notions of pharmacology and pharmacognosy; preparation of homemade forms; toxicity; notions of health surveillance, indications and contraindications.

This type of therapy is so widespread in the city of Vitória that more than 110 physicians across the network of primary care often prescribe these drugs. With these physicians, a survey was made in 2003 by Municipal Health Secretary about the satisfaction with the use of herbal medicines, which resulted in meaningful indicators: 70% considered good results, 54% were satisfied with the herbal medicine, 93% considered good user acceptance.

Since 1997 there has been a growth of 110% in the number of prescritions for herbal medicines. Only in 2002 16,918 formulations were prepared of a total of 11,138 prescriptions served in the city.

There is strict technical criteria for the drugs to reach the users with quality. In Vitória, Pharmacies in the Basic Health Unit/ Health Family you can find the following herbal products: *Achillea millefolium* L., *Ageratum conyzoides* L., *Baccharis trimera* Mart.,

Calendula officinalis L., *Verbenaceae Cordia* D.C. *Erytrina mulungu*, *Matricaria recutita* L. *Maytenus ilicifolia* Mart. *Melissa officinalis* L., *Mikania giomerata* Spreg., *Passiflora edulis*, *Phyllanthus niruri*, *Plantago major* L. (Brasil, 2008d).

4. The implementation of the National Policy of Integrative and Complementary Practices (PNPIC): Goals and challenges

Due to the absence of specific guidelines, the experiences conducted in state and municipal public network have occurred in an unequal and discontinued manner and often without due registration, adequate supply of inputs, or follow up and assessment actions. Based on the current experiences, the PNPIC defines the approaches of the Traditional Medicine and Complementary/Alternative Medicine in the SUS considering also the increasing legitimacy of such experiences by society.

According to the PNPIC (Brasil, 2006a; Brazil, 2008) objectives of the Policy are:

• To incorporate and implement the Traditional Medicine and Complementary/Alternative Medicine in the SUS, in the perspective of injury prevention and the promotion and recovery of health, with emphasis in the basic attention, for the continuous humanized and integral health care.
• To contribute for the increase of the System resolubility and broader access to the Traditional Medicine and Complementary/Alternative Medicine, ensuring quality, effectiveness, efficiency and safety in its use.
• To promote the rationalization of health actions, stimulating innovative and socially contributive alternatives to the sustainable development of the communities.
• To stimulate actions regarding the social control/ participation, promoting the responsible and continuous involvement of the users, managers and professionals in the different instances of health policies effectiveness.

Some points still represent major challenges. Overcoming these challenges will depend essentially on the prioritization of the Traditional Medicine and Complementary/Alternative Medicine in government plans and the coordination between civil society and the health system. Among the main challenges listed below are considered the most immediate and strategic development the PNPIC in the SUS:

• Viability of training and qualification of professionals in adequate numbers, to work with Traditional Medicine and Complementary/Alternative Medicine;
• Implementation Monitoring and Evaluation, considering the general policy guidelines, the institutionalization of the evaluation of primary care, the specifics of each component and system levels;
• Provision of material resources (homeopathic / herbal medicines, needles for Traditional Chinese Medicine/acupuncture);
• Implementation of Research in Traditional Medicine and Complementary/Alternative Medicine, encouraging the expansion of knowledge, considering the needs and SUS guidelines, among others (Simoni et al., 2008).

Rosa et al. (2011) pointed out that it is not enough governments to institute Traditional Medicine and Complementary/Alternative Medicine or even law enacted to ensure that they offer quality, it is necessary to promote opportunities for discussion in both academic spaces and services, considering the difficulties to use a "new" paradigm of health care.

5. Final considerations

In this chapter only some experience of Traditional Medicine and Complementary/Alternative Medicine in health services could be described. However, there are in all regions in all 26 states and the Federal District of the Federative Republic of Brazil, experiences being developed on this topic (Brasil, 2008a; Brasil, 2008b; Brasil, 2008c; Brasil, 2008d; Brasil, 2008e; Brasil, 2008f; Brasil 2008g). Such experiences can serve as references for health services that ensure the universality in the SUS.

The introduction of the Integrative and Complementary Practices in the Primary Health Care seek the improvement of the services provided as well as the number of different approaches in the process of delivering health. Public health policies coupled with the WHO encouragement materialize such a priority, revealing the necessary safety, efficacy, and quality from the perspective of integral health care. Not many countries have national policies for traditional medicine. Regulating traditional medicine products, practices and practitioners is difficult due to variations in definitions and categorizations of traditional medicine therapies. A single herbal product could be defined as either a food, a dietary supplement or an herbal medicine, depending on the country. This disparity in regulations at the national level has implications for international access and distribution of products (WHO, 2005).

It is observed that the institutionalization of Integrative and Complementary Practices in Brazil has been a historically built process. It was the result of years of debate on the topic and involved both the scientific community and civic society.

The SUS was created in 1990. After 20 years of its creation, is in a consolidation process. The insertion of Traditional Medicine and Complementary/Alternative Medicine system is contemplating the doctrinal principles of SUS (universality, equity and integrality) and helps to strengthen the system, which is a social victory of the Brazilian people.

6. References

Araújo, E. C. (2008). Homeopathy: an approach to the subject in the process of diseasing. *Ciência & saúde coletiva*, Vol. 13, suppl., (Abril/2008), pp. 663-671, ISSN 1413-8123

Associação Comunitária Monte Azul/SP (2011). Saúde. 25.10.2011. Available from <http://www.sab.org.br/monteazul/>

Aune, A.; Alraek, T.; LiHua, H. & Baerheim, A. (1998). Acupuncture in the prophylaxis of recurrent lower urinary tract infection in adult women. *Scandinavian Journal of Primary Health Care*, Vol. 16, No 1, (March/1998), pp. 37-39, ISSN 0281-3432

Ballegaard, S.; Pedersen, F.; Pietersen, A.; Nissen V. H & Olsen N. V. (1990). Effects of acupuncture in moderate, stable angina pectoris: a controlled study. *Journal of Internal Medicine*, Vol. 227, No 1, (January/1990), pp. 25-30, ISSN 0954-6820

Blumenthal, M. (Ed). (1998). *The complet German comission E monographs: therapeutic guide to herbal medicines.* American Botanical Council, ISBN 0-9655555-0-X, Austin, United State of America

Brasil. (1986). *8ªConferência Nacional de Saúde, 17 a 21 de março de 1986.* 25.10.2011. Available from: <http://conselho.saude.gov.br/biblioteca/Relatorios/relatorio_8.pdf>

Brasil. (1990). *Lei n° 8.080, de 19 de setembro de 1990.* 26.10.2011. Available from: < http://portal.saude.gov.br/portal/arquivos/pdf/lei8080.pdf>

Brasil. (1998a). *Relatório final da 10 ° Conferência Nacional de Saúde,Brasília-DF, 2 a 6 de setembro de 1996.* Ministério da Saúde, ISBN 85-334-0173-6, Brasília, Brasil

Brasil. (1998b). Ministério da Saúde. *Portaria n° 3916/MS/GM, de 30 de outubro de 1998*. 20.10.2011. Available from: <http://www.anvisa.gov.br/legis/consolidada/portaria_3916_98.pdf>

Brasil. (2003). *12° Conferência Nacional de Saúde: Conferência Sergio Arouca: Brasília 7 a 11 de dezembro de 2003: Relatório Final*. Ministério da Saúde/ Conselho Nacional de Saúde, ISBN 85-334-0816-1, Brasília, Brasil

Brasil. (2004a). Conselho Nacional de Saúde. *Resolução CNS n° 338, de 06 de maio de 2004*. 25.10.2011. Available from: <http://portal.saude.gov.br/portal/arquivos/pdf/resol_cns338.pdf

Brasil. (2004b). Conselho Nacional de Saúde. *Resolução CNS n° 343, de 07 de outubro de 2004*. 25.10.2011. Available from: <http://www.conselho.saude.gov.br/resolucoes/reso_04.htm>

Brasil. (2005). *Conferência Nacional de Medicamentos e Assistência Farmacêutica: Relatório Final: efetivando o acesso a qualidade e a humanização na assistência farmacêutica com controle social*. Ministério da Saúde/ Conselho Nacional de Saúde, ISBN 85-334-0848-X, Brasília, Brasil

Brasil. (2006a). Ministério da Saúde. Secretaria de Atenção à Saúde. Departamento de Atenção Básica. *Política Nacional de Práticas Integrativas e Complementares no SUS-PNPIC-SUS*. Ministério da Saúde, ISBN 85-334-1208-8, Brasília, Brasil

Brasil. (2006b). Ministério da Saúde. Secretaria de Ciência, Tecnologia e Insumo Estratégicos. Departamento de Assistência Farmacêutica. *Política Nacional de Plantas Medicinais e fitoterápicos*. Ministério da Saúde, ISBN 85-334-1042-1, Brasília, Brasil

Brasil. (2008a). Ministério da Saúde. Medicina Antroposófica a serviço do ser humano. *Revista Brasileira Saúde da Família*, Ed. Especial (Maio/2008), pp. 44-49, ISSN 1518-2355

Brasil. (2008b). Ministério da Saúde. João Del Rei prova que tradição é uma conquista e luta por manter a medicina antroposófica. *Revista Brasileira Saúde da Família*, Ed. Especial (Maio/2008), pp. 47-49, ISSN 1518-2355

Brasil. (2008c). Ministério da Saúde. Lian Gong: uma conquista coletiva no interior de São Paulo. *Revista Brasileira Saúde da Família*, Ed. Especial (Maio/2008), pp. 35-37, ISSN 1518-2355

Brasil. (2008d). Ministério da Saúde. Vitória: Fitoterapia nas Unidades Básicas de Saúde. *Revista Brasileira Saúde da Família*, Ed. Especial (Maio/2008), pp. 50-53, ISSN 1518-2355

Brasil. (2008e). Ministério da Saúde. Terapias integrativas fazem história em Campinas. *Revista Brasileira Saúde da Família*, Ed. Especial (Maio/2008), pp. 20-25, ISSN 1518-2355

Brasil. (2008f). Ministério da Saúde. Amapá conta com centro de referência para toda a região norte. *Revista Brasileira Saúde da Família*, Ed. Especial (Maio/2008), pp. 30-34, ISSN 1518-2355

Brasil. (2008g). Ministério da Saúde. Acupuntura e Fitoterapia no acompanhamento do climatério. *Revista Brasileira Saúde da Família*, Ed. Especial (Maio/2008), pp. 54-57, ISSN 1518-2355

Brasil. (2011). Instituto Brasileiro de Geográfica e Estatística. *Sinopse do censo brasileiro 2010*. Ministério do Planejamento, Orçamento e Gestão, ISBN 978-85-240-4187-7, Rio de Janeiro, Brasil

Brazil. (2008). Ministry of Health of Brazil. Secretary of Health Care. Department of Primary Care. *PNPIC: National Policy on Integrative and Complementary Practices of the SUS: access expansion initiative*, Ministry of Health of Brazil, ISBN 978-85-334-1462-4, Brasília, Brazil

Bullock, M. L; Culliton, P. D. & Olander, R. T. (1989). Controlled trial of acupuncture for severe recidivist alcoholism. *Lancet*, Vol. 1, No 8652, (June/1989), pp. 1435-1439, ISSN 0140-6736

Centers for Disease Control and Prevention (2011). *Dengue*, 13.08.2011, Available from <http://www.cdc.gov/dengue/>

Conselho Federal de Medicina (1980). *Resolução CFM n° 1000/1980,* 25.10.2011. Available from < http://www.portalmedico.org.br/resolucoes/cfm/1989/1000_1989.htm>

Conselho Federal de Medicina (1993). *Parecer Técnico n° 21, de 23 de novembro de 1993,* 25.10.2011. Available from < http://www.portalmedico.org.br/pareceres/CFM/1993/21_1993.htm>

David, J.; Modi, S.; Aluko, A. A.; Robertshaw, C. & Farebrother, J. (1998). Chronic neck pain: a comparison of acupuncture treatment and physiotherapy. *British Journal of Rheumatology,* Vol. 37, No 10, (October/1998), pp. 1118-1132, ISSN 0263-7103

Diehl, D. L. Acupuncture for gastrointestinal and hepatobiliary disorders. (1999). *Journal of Alternative and Complementary Medicine,* Vol. 5, No 1, (February/1999), pp. 27-45, ISSN 1075-5335

Dundee, J. W.; Ghaly, R. G.; Fitzpatrick, K. T.; Lynch, G. A. & Abram, W. P. (1987). Acupuncture to prevent cisplatin-associated vomiting. *Lancet,* Vol. 1, No 8541, (May/1987), pp. 1083, ISSN 0140-6736

Ferreira, C. S. & Luz, M.T. (2007). Shen: structuring category in the rationale of Chinese medical. *História, Ciência, Saúde-Manguinhos,* Vol. 14, No. 3 (Setembro/2007), pp. 863-875, ISSN 0104-5970

Jobst, K.; Chen, J.H.; McPherson, K.; Arrowsmith, J.; Brown, V.; Efthimiou, J.; Fletcher, H.J. et al. (1986). Controlled trial of acupuncture for disabling breathlessness. *Lancet,* Vol. 2, No 8521-8522, (December/1986), pp. 1416-1419, ISSN 0140-6736

Joshi, Y. M. (1992). Acupuncture in bronchial asthma. *Journal of the Association of Physicians of India,* Vol. 40, No 5, (May/1992), pp. 327-331, ISSN 0004-5772

Lao, L.; Bergman, S.; Langenberg, P.; Wong, R. H. & Berman, B. (1995). Efficacy of Chinese acupuncture on postoperative oral surgery pain. *Oral Surgery, Oral Medicine, Oral Pathology, Oral Radiology and Endodontics,* Vol. 79, No 4, (April/1995), pp. 423-428, ISSN 1079-2104

Lee, M. L.(2006). *Lian Gong em 18 Terapias - Forjando um Corpo Saudável: Ginástica Chinesa do Dr. Zhuang Yuen Ming,* Pensamentos, ISBN 85-315-1024-4, São Paulo, Brasil

Lee, Y. H.; Lee, W. C.;, Chen, M. T.; Huang, J. K.; Chung, C. & Chang, L. S. (1992).Acupuncture in the treatment of renal colic. *Journal of Urology,* Vol. 147, No 1, (January/1992), pp. 16-18, ISSN 0022-5347

Luz, M. T. (2005). Contemporary culture and complementary medicine: new paradigm in health in the end of the century. *Physis,* Vol.15, suppl., (Junho/2005), pp. 145-176, ISSN 0103-7331

Matos, F.J. (1998). *Farmácias vivas: sistema de utilização de plantas medicinais projetado para pequenas comunidades.* Editora da Universidade Federal do Ceára, ISBN 85-7282-008-6, Fortaleza, Brazil

Marino, R. (2008). Homeopathy and collective health: the case of dengue epidemics. *International Journal of High Dilution Research,* Vol. 7, No. 25 (December/2008), pp. 179-185, ISSN 1982-6206

Nunes, L. A. S. (2008). Contribution of homeopathy to the control of an outbreak of dengue in Macaé, Rio de Janeiro. *International Journal of High Dilution Research,* Vol. 7, No. 25 (December/2008), pp. 186-192, ISSN 1982-6206

Petrie, J. P. & Hazleman, B. L. (1986). A controlled study of acupuncture in neck pain. *British Journal of Rheumatology,* Vol. 25, No 3, (August/1986), pp. 271-275, ISSN 0263-7103

Rosa, C.; Câmara, S. G. & Béria, J. U. (2011). Representations and use intention of phytoterapy in primary health care. *Ciência & saúde coletiva*, Vol. 16, No. 1, (Janeiro/2011), pp. 311-318, ISSN 1413-8123

Secretaria da Saúde do Estado de Goiás/Brazil. (September 2011a). *Hospital de Medicina Alternativa-HMA*, 27.09.2011, Available from <http://www.saude.go.gov.br/index.php?idEditoria=4129>

Secretaria da Saúde do Estado de Goiás/Brazil. (October 2011b). *Hospital de Medicina Alternativa-Uma experiência a ser compartilhada*, 13.10.2011, Available from <http://www.sgc.goias.gov.br/upload/links/arq_285_hma23anos.pdf>

Simoni, C.; Benevides, I. & Barros, N. F. (2008). As Práticas Integrativas e Complementares no SUS: realidade e desafios após dois anos de publicação da PNPIC. *Revista Brasileira Saúde da Família*, Ed. Especial (Maio/2008), pp. 70-76, ISSN 1518-2355

Vincent, C.A. (1989). A controlled trial of the treatment of migraine by acupuncture. *The Clinical Journal of Pain*, Vol. 5, No 4, (December/1989), pp. 305-312, ISSN 0749-8047

Vilholm, O. J.; Møller, K. & Jørgensen, K. (1998). Effect of traditional Chinese acupuncture on severe tinnitus: a double-blind, placebo-controlled clinical investigation with open therapeutic control. *British Journal of Audiology*, Vol. 32, No 3, (June/1998), pp. 197-204, ISSN 0300-5364

Washburn, A.M.; Fullilove, R. E.; Fullilove, M. T.; Keenan, P. A.; McGee, B.; Morris, K. A.; Sorensen, J. L. & Clark, W. W (1993). Acupuncture heroin detoxification: a single-blind clinical trial. *Journal of Substance Abuse Treatment*, Vol. 10, No 4, (July - August/1993), pp. 345-351, ISSN 0740-5472

Wong, A. M.; Su, T. Y.; Tang, F.T.; Cheng, P.T. & Liaw, M.Y. (1999). Clinical trial of electrical acupuncture on hemiplegic stroke patients. *American Journal of Physical Medicine and Rehabilitation*, Vol. 78, No 2, (March/1999), pp. 117-122, ISSN 0894-9115

World Health Organization/ United Nations Childrens Fund. (1978). *Primary health care : report of the International Conference on Primary Health Care, Alma-Ata, USSR, 6-12 September 1978*, "Health for all" series, No.1. WHO, ISBN 92 4 180001 1, Geneva, Switzerland

World Health Organization. (1999). *WHO monographs on selected medicinal plants*. WHO, ISBN 92 4 154517 7 WHO, ISBN 92 4 154543 7, Geneva, Switzerland

World Health Organization. (2002a). *WHO Traditional Medicine Strategy 2002-2005*, WHO, Retrieved from: < http://whqlibdoc.who.int/hq/2002/who_edm_trm_2002.1.pdf>

World Health Organization. (2002b). *WHO monographs on selected medicinal plants*. WHO, ISBN 92 4 154537 2, Geneva, Switzerland

World Health Organization. (2003). *Acupuncture: review and analysis of reports on controlled trials*. WHO, ISBN 92 4 154543 7, Geneva, Switzerland

World Health Organization. (2005). *National policy on traditional medicine and regulation of herbal medicines: Report of a WHO global survey*. WHO, ISBN 92 4 159323 7, Geneva, Switzerland

World Health Organization. (2009). *Dengue: guidelines for diagnosis, treatment, prevetion and control*. WHO, ISBN 978 92 4 154787 1, Geneva, Switzerland

World Health Organization. (2011). *The world medicines situations 2011. Traditional medicines: global situation, issues and challenges*, WHO, Retrieved from: <http://www.who.int/medicines/areas/policy/world_medicines_situation/WMS_ch18_wTraditionalMed.pdf >

9

Skills in Minor Surgical Procedures for General Practitioners

Jose María Arribas Blanco and María Hernández Tejero
Faculty of Medicine, Autonomous University of Madrid, Madrid, Spain

1. Introduction

Minor surgery is defined as a set of procedures in which short surgical techniques are applied on superficial tissues. Local anaesthesia is often required for these procedures and their complication-rate as well as the risk involved is low.

Lesions and problems requiring these procedures for diagnostic or therapeutical reasons are frequently seen by general practitioners both in the outpatient setting (excision of skin lesions, for instance) as well as in the emergency care setting (wound suturing, for example). Therefore, for family doctors proficiency in minor surgical procedures is an additional tool for good medical practice and acquiring skills in minor surgical procedures has become a critical part of medical training, and has adjusted their professional profile to the problems and needs arising in te daily practice of family medicine.

Achieving clinical excellence in these procedures depends on the involved practitioner's level of technical training, since surgical training is the best way to learn the correct surgical gestures and proper use of surgical instruments. Trainees must also understand that a sound diagnostic approach plus the observance of basic principles of good medical practice are prerequisites for clinical excellence in their practice of minor surgical procedures

It is shown that the performance of minor surgery in primary care is good for patients, for health care system and for the practitioner; In addition to being fun and rewarding. However, those procedures are not without risks, both during surgery and afterwards. Therefore, any surgical procedure performed by the family physician, is necessary (in addition to proper surgical technique and appropriate therapeutic indications) provide a comprehensive, clear and complete information to the patient, which will be reflected with the Informed Consent signed by the patient before carrying out any minor surgical intervention.The realization of Informed Consent is not a guarantee of exculpate in the event of a judicial proceeding by a complaint from a medical act of minor surgery. The judge will assess good medical practice and clinical experience based on the *lex artis* (proper patient selection and indications for its implementation, use of good surgical technique ..). Therefore, and although the academic programs of the Family Medicine Specialty explicitly enable the family doctor to perform minor surgical procedures, it is recommended that primary care physicians have medical insurance with specific coverage for surgical techniques.

This chapter will try and help general practitioners master minor surgical procedures by answering the following questions:

1. Where should general practitioners perform minor surgical procedures?
   Optimal infrastructure and medical furniture for a Minor Surgery operating room and doctor's preparation
2. Which are the instruments and materials involved?
   Surgical instruments (plus their handling) and suture materials for basic and advanced surgery.
3. How to perform minor surgical procedures in the primary care setting?
   Anaesthesia techniques: local anaesthetic infiltration and regional blocks
   Basic and Advanced Surgical Techniques in Minor Surgery
4. Preoperative considerations
   Body areas of risk in minor surgery. Basic knowledge of the topographic anatomy of the skin. The most common pathologies in minor surgery: diagnostic criteria
5. Performance of the surgical procedure
   Elliptical excision
6. Good clinical practice in minor surgery and complications in minor surgery.

2. The minor surgery room and physician's preparation

2.1 The minor surgery room

Minor surgical procedures do not involve very sophisticated devices. However, some basic requirements in terms of infrastructure and equipment must be met[1,2].

Although some minor surgical procedures could be performed in a consulting room or office in the primary care setting, it is recommended that each facility has a specific room for these procedures. This room (Fig 1) must include:

Surgical room: a well-ventilated, square or rectangular, 15-20 square- meter room is necessary, with a suitable temperature and a good source of artificial light. It is imperative that it is clean, but it does not require sterile isolation. The surgical room should be cleaned properly at the end of the surgical session, particularly after contaminated procedures (e.g. abscesses). Having a room exclusively dedicated to surgical procedures is ideal, but a well-equipped treatment room is acceptable. It is advisable to have a sink with a mixer tap control plus an automatic soap applicator for hand washing.

Operating table: it should be located in the centre of the room to allow easy access from both sides. Height-adjustable, articulated tables are preferred. It should be of washable material. In any case, it is essential to have a table that allows the doctor to work in comfort, both standing and sitting. Low beds used for physical examination are not acceptable, since doctors will be forced to work in awkward positions.

Doctor's stool: long procedures are best performed in a sitting position. A height-adjustable stool on wheels is, therefore, necessary.

Side Table: it is used to place the surgical instruments and material used during the surgery. It must have wheels and be height- adjustable, and it should be placed near the surgical field, facilitating the procedure. Placing surgical material on the patient must be avoided, to prevent it from falling in case the patient moves during the procedure.

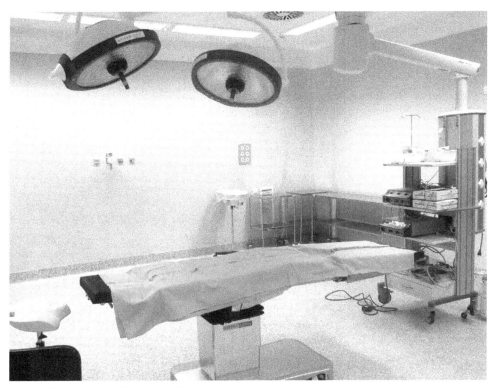

Fig. 1. Well-equipped Room of Minor Surgery.

Lamp: it must provide adequate lighting with, at least, 45,000 lux of iluminance. Lamps may be fixed to the wall or ceiling of the room but portable lamps with wheels are also acceptable. These lamps can be moved in several directions, their light intensity cam be modulated and their spotlight can be focused. It is advisable to have another auxiliary lamp with a magnifying glass, which will be useful for removing foreign bodies or working under magnification.

Showcase and containers: some space should also be left for storing consumables and surgical instruments. There should also be properly marked containers for bio contaminated material, and a disposal system in accordance with current health legislation.

Resuscitation equipment: although life-threatening events are extremely rare in minor surgery, it is nonetheless essential to have a crash trolley with cardiopulmonary resuscitation equipment, including material for vascular access, airway intubation, saline, drugs for resuscitation (e.g. epinephrine, atropine, bicarbonate) and a defibrillator.

Sterilization system: any medical facility performing surgical procedures must have an autoclave to sterilize surgical equipment or set up an external circuit to sterilize the material.

2.2 Physician's preparation for minor surgery

Performing minor surgical procedures carries some risk of transmission of infectious diseases (such as HCV and HIV), both from patient to doctor and vice versa. To minimize this risk, universal precautions should be adopted and applied by all physicians performing invasive procedures to any patient regardless of their serological status. These measures include the use of appropriate clothing and accessories and proper hand washing as well as sterile technique for surgical glove placement.

Surgical attire: In minor surgical procedures we consider essential the use of surgical shirts and trousers ("scrubs") or gowns and sterile gloves. The use of surgical masks and eye goggles is considered highly desirable. Disposable gowns are very useful.

Hand washing: There are different methods of surgical scrubbing. Hygienic scrubbing involves using a normal soap solution (no brush) and washing thoroughly all skin folds for at least 20 seconds and is appropriate for all minor surgical procedures. Anatomic scrubbing is left for major surgery.

Time span from scrubbing to glove placement should never exceed 10 minutes.

Sterile glove placement: surgical gloves are sterile and single use and are available in various sizes. Some manufacturers use a numerical sizing (from 6 ½ to 8 ½) while others use an alphanumeric sizing (XS, S, M, L, XL). There are models with and without latex as well as powder-free models.

Glove placement should be completed without contaminating the outer surface of the glove, i.e. the inner or powdered part of the glove can be touched with the hands, while the outer or non- powdered surface should only be touched with the other glove.

Unquestionably, gloves act as a barrier against body fluids from accidental cuts or punctures. In some surgeries with increased risk of glove perforation the use of double gloves is recommended, because it decreases the risk of perforation and, therefore, the risk of patient to doctor contamination.

3. Surgical instruments (handling) and suture material

3.1 surgical instruments for minor surgery

General practitioners should have a thorough knowledge of surgical instruments, including their handling and maintenance. The quality, condition and type of instruments used in any procedure can affect its outcome. Choosing the right instruments for each surgical intervention is, therefore, an important issue[1].

In the following paragraphs we will briefly describe the main features of the instruments recommended for minor surgical procedures.

Scalpel: it allows the surgeon to cut with precision through the skin and other tissues and is also used for non-blunt dissection.

A number 3 handle with number 11 and 15 blades must be available. The scalpel blade is installed on the handlle in a unique position, matching the blade guide with the handle guide. The scalpel is handled with the dominant hand like a pencil (fig. 2), allowing small and precise incisions. The hand should be partially supported on the working surface to increase precision. Using the contralateral hand the skin should be tightened perpendicularly to the direction of the incision. The blade should cut the skin perpendicularly (bevelled incisions should be avoided), except in hairy areas (scalp or eyebrows) where the incision should be parallel to the hairshafts, to avoid damaging the follicles.

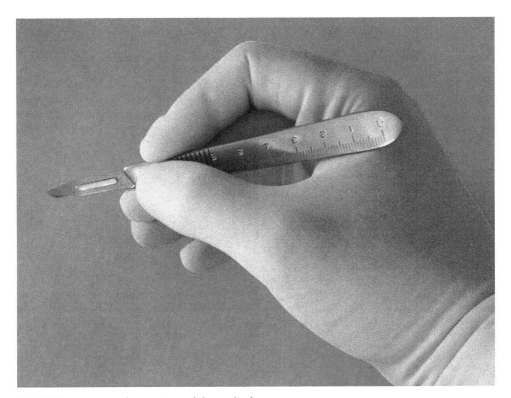

Fig. 2. Correct way of managing of the scalpel

Scissors: they are used both for cutting or sectioning tissues and different materials such as sutures, drains, and bandages, and dissecting through different tissues.

A 14 cm. long curved blunt May scissors (cutting scissors) and an 11.5 cm curved blunt Metzenbaum scissors (dissecting scissors) should be available. The use of dissecting scissors for cutting materials is not recommended.

Scissors are handled by inserting part of the distal phalanges of the thumb and fourth finger into the rings, and then supporting the second finger on the branches of the instrument. For blunt dissection (using Metzenbaum scissors), scissors are inserted with the tip closed and are then opened, separating the tissues in more or less anatomical layers. For sharp dissection scissors are inserted with the tip open and the blades are then closed, cutting the tissue.

Dissection manoeuvres should be performed gently and with a good exposure of the surgical field, never in a blind fashion, to avoid irreversible damage to anatomical structures. To this aim, it is essential to know the topographic anatomy of the operative site.

Needle-holder: needle-holders are meant to hold curved needles while stitching.Their jaws are especially designed to hold needles safely and atraumatically. The needle is held 2/3 of the way back from its point. A small or medium (12 to 15 cm.) standard needle holder with a tip suitable for needles up to 4/0 is recommended. Long needle holders are not recommended for minor surgeries.

Like other instruments with rings, the needle holder is handled by inserting a portion of the distal phalanges of the thumb and fourth finger of the dominant hand into the rings, while the index finger is directed towards the tip of the instrument (Fig 3). When performing the suture, the needle holder should describe a prono-supination movement to facilitate the passage of the needle through the tissues. The angle of entry of the needle into the skin should be 90 ° for a proper edge eversion of the wound. The non-dominant hand holds the skin with a dissecting forceps or a retractor, to oppose the pressure of the needle

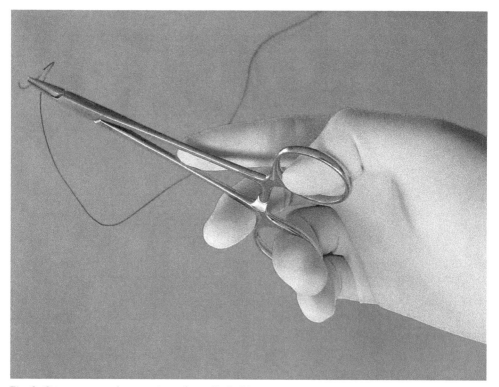

Fig. 3. Correct way of managing of needle-holders

Dissecting Forceps: Use of a 12 cm- long Adson forceps with teeth to handle the skin, plus a toothless Adson forceps for suture removal is recommended. If Adson forceps are not available, they may be replaced by two standard forceps, one with and one without teeth. It is important not to manipulate the skin using non-toothed forceps.

Used with the nondominant hand, forceps are the most important auxiliary instrument. They allow the surgeon to expose the tissues that are to be incised, dissected and sutured, while the other hand uses the main surgical instrument. Forceps are handled similar to holding a pencil, between the first, second and third fingers.

Haemostats: 2 or 3 12 cm curved non-toothed Mosquito forceps must be available. Haemostats are used to pull tissue, for haemostasis and, in some cases, for blunt dissection in absence of small scissors. Haemostats are handled by inserting the thumb and fourth finger through the rings, while the second finger is directed towards the tip of the instrument.

Although a basic set of surgical instruments (including the previously described instruments [Fig 4]) is enough for most minor surgical interventions, certain surgical procedures require familiarity with the use of especial instruments or equipment such as curettes, punches, the bovie, or surgical retractors.

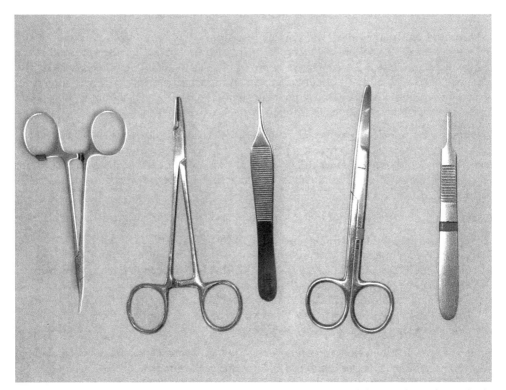

Fig. 4. Basic Set of instruments of minor surgery: scalpel (handle of the number 3 for scalpel number 15), scissors of May, Adson forceps with teeth, needle-holders and Mosquito forceps

Surgical retractors: these instruments are used to expose the surgical field through separation or retraction of the edges of the wound. If an assistant is available, he or she will hold the retractors. Otherwise, the surgeon will hold the retractor in his/her non dominant hand. In minor surgery, it is advisable to have a Senn-Mueller retractor (which is also called double-end retractor, due to its having a wide plate on one side and three sharp hooks on the other). Another useful retractor for delicate surgery is the simple skin hook.

Biopsy punch: it is an instrument consisting of a handle and a cylindrical cutting edge (trephine) for obtaining tissue biopsies. They are usually disposable and are manufactured in different diameters (2 to 8 mm), the most useful in minor surgery being the 4 mm punch. These instruments allow the surgeon to obtain full- thickness samples of the skin. They are handled with the dominant hand, performing rotational movements of the instrument to cut the skin and obtain the sample[3].

Curette: it is an instrument consisting of a handle and a spoon-shaped or cutting ring end that allows scraping of lesions on the skin surface. They can be disposable or not, and they are manufactured in different diameters. The curette is handled with the dominant hand using a simple surgical technique that involves "scraping" or enucleating different types of superficial, hyperkeratotic or raised partial-thickness skin lesions.

Cryosurgical equipment: these are devices that spray a cryogen, which is usually liquid nitrogen to treat skin lesions. The cryogen may also be applied by using a swab[4]. The cryogen is stored in tanks or containers to prevent its evaporation (Fig 5). There are mobile units equipped with a nitrogen- spraying mechanism, which are endowed with a range of nozzles and probes that allow the surgeon to control the intensity of the spray, depending on the dimensions and location of the lesion that needs to be treated.

Electrocautery: the electrocautery or bovie is an electrical device consisting of a central unit that applies an electric current through a sterile terminal with capacity to coagulate and cut through different tissues. It also consists of a ground to close the electrical circuit (Fig 6). There are different terminals depending on the type of procedure that is to be performed[5].

A set of surgical instruments for minor surgical procedures should include:

- One 14-16 cm-long standard needle holder (Webster, Crile-Wood, Hegar)
- Two curved non-toothed Mosquito hemostats
- One 14 cm-long standard dissecting forceps or 1 Adson dissecting forceps with teeth
- One 14 cm-long standard non-toothed dissecting forceps
- One scalpel handle # 3, with No. 15 disposable blades
- One 14 cm-long curved or straight blunt May scissors
- One 14 cm-long curved blunt Metzenbaum scissors

Optional: 1 or 2 double-end retractors (Senn-Muller), and a sterile marker. An optimal allocation should include electrosurgical and cryosurgical equipment

Care of surgical instruments

Surgical instruments are expensive. With proper care, an instrument should last ten years or more. Eventually instruments deteriorate through normal use, but most of the damage is due to improper cleaning and handling. On the other hand, instruments should always be used in sterile conditions since minor surgical procedures require sterilization of all surgical material. In accordance, the following guidelines should be respected:

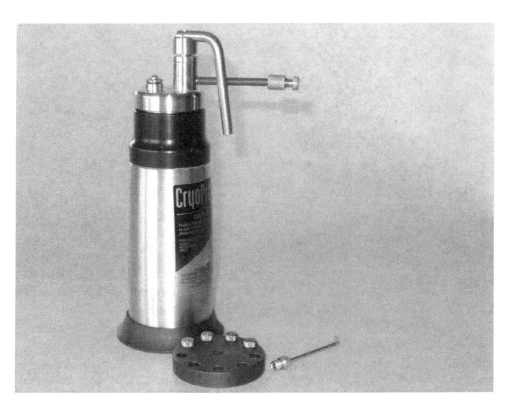

Fig. 5. Equipo de criocirugía. Portable unit of cryosurgery for liquid nitrogen. It consists of a thermos of stainless steel, covered with a structure of bronze and stainless steel, with a special system of valves and a great mouth of filling, the pulverization being controlled by means of a trigger. They are light and of easy transport.

- Separate (using gloves) single-use sharps and throw them in the container for biocontaminated material.
- Do not place the instruments in saline, which can deteriorate the instruments and do not allow organic matter to dry on the instruments after use. Instruments should be placed into a container with some disinfecting solution (glutaraldehyde phenolate, disinfecting solution of phenol, sodium tetraborate, glutaraldehyde or 0.05% chlorhexidine solution).
- Sterilize. The most appropriate method is using an autoclave with quality control of the sterilization process

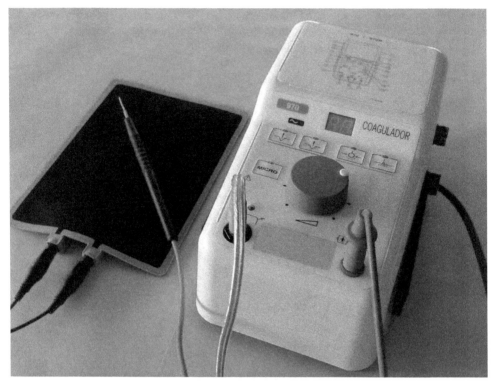

Fig. 6. Unit of electrobisturí, terminal and capture of land.

3.2 Suture materials

Different types of suture materials are available: threads, staples, adhesive sutures and tissue adhesives. The use of a particular suture material or a particular type of needle can make a difference in surgical outcome. Suture choice should be based on scientific criteria, and tempered by good practical experience.

Thread sutures provide a secure wound closure and ensure the strongest wound- support and minimal wound- dehiscence rate compared to other types of closure[6,7], but require the use of anesthesia, operating time is increased, tissue is traumatized, foreign bodies are inserted in the wound and the risk of disease transmission by accidental inoculation is increased.

Conventional sutures may be replaced by mechanical sutures, which reduce surgical time or by adhesive tapes, which provide lower reactivity and a lower infection rate, as previously mentioned. Tissue glues or adhesives arise in this context as an alternative to the usual procedures[8].

Sutures

They are classified according to their origin (natural, such as silk, or synthetic polymers that produce less tissue reaction), their configuration (monofilament or multifilament), their size (the thickness of the suture is measured using a zero-scale [USP system] with more zeros meaning finer sutures) (fig 7). The most commonly used in minor surgery range from 2 / 0 to 4 / 0 or 5 / 0, the finest sutures are usually attached to smaller needles and require the use of more precise needle holders.

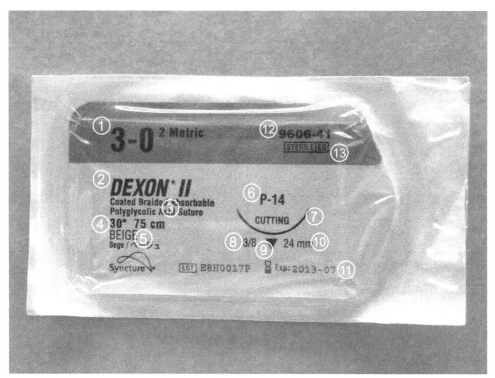

Fig. 7. Information of on of suture: (1) calibre of the thread (system USP and metric), (2) trade name of the suture, (3) composition and physical structure of the thread, (4) length of the thread, (5) color of the thread, (6) model of needle (every manufacturer uses different references), (7) I draw from the needle to scale 1:1, (8) circumference of the needle (expressed in parts of circle), (9) section of the needle, (10) length of the needle, (11) expiry date, (12) indexes of the manufacturer, (13) indicator of sterile packing.

The size and type of suture will be selected depending on the anatomical site, the type of wound and on the patient's features (Table 1).

Features of main sutures

Nonabsorbable sutures: They are not degraded by the body (or their degradation process is very slowly). They are used for skin wounds in which stitches that are to be removed or for internal structures that must maintain a constant tension (like tendons and ligaments):

1. Silk: Suitable for skin suture and for removable sutures in general, although it may cause significant tissue reaction.

2. Nylon: Indicated for precise skin sutures and internal structures that must maintain constant tension (e.g. tendons). Nylon is more difficult to handle but it causes minimal tissue reaction
3. Polypropylene: Indicated in continuous intradermal skin closure. It is a very soft suture with high package memory and, therefore, it requires more knots for secure tying. Polypropylene causes minimal tissue reaction

Anatomical region	Skin suturing	Subcutaneous suturing (whenever necessary)	Stitch removal	
			Adults	children
scalp	staples 2/0 silk	Vicryl® or Dexon® 3/0	7-9	6-8
eyelids	6/0 monofilament 6/0 silk	-	3-5	3-5
ears	4/0-5/0 monofilament 4/0-5/0 silk	-	4-5	3-5
nose	4/0 monofilament 4/0 silk	Vicryl® or Dexon® 4/0	4-6	3-5
lips	4/0 monofilament 4/0 silk	Vicryl® or Dexon® 4/0	4-6	4-5
Forehead and face neck	4/0-5/0 monofilament 4/0-5/0 silk	Vicryl® or Dexon® 4/0	4-6	3-5
Trunk / abdomen	3/0-4/0 monofilament	Vicryil® or Dexon® 3/0	7-12	7-9
back	3/0-4/0 monofilament	Vicryil® or Dexon® 3/0	12-14	14
Upper limb / hand	4/0 monofilament	Vicryil® or Dexon® 3/0	8-10	7-9
Pulp of fingers	4/0 monofilament	-	10-12	8-10
Lower extremity	3/0 monofilament staples	Vicryil® or Dexon® 3/0	8-12	7-10
foot	4/0 monofilament	Vicryil® or Dexon® 3/0	10-12	8-10
penis	4/0 monofilament	Vicryil® or Dexon® 3/0	7-10	6-8
Mouth and tongue	3/0 Vicryil®	-	-	-

Table 1. Indications of types of sutures and time for stitch removal

Absorbable Sutures: A suture is considered absorbable if, when placed under the skin surface, it loses most of its tensile strength in 60 days. Complete resorption is, thus, not required for a suture to be considered absorbable. These sutures gradually disappear from the body by biological absorption or hydrolysis, causing an inflammatory reaction in the body. Absorbable sutures are use for deep or non-removable suturing.

1. Polyglactin 910: Indicated in dermal suturing, subcutaneous tissue, deep suturing and ligatures of small vessels.
2. Polyglycolic acid: its indications are similar to the previous

Stitch removal

The lapse of time (in days) recommended for the removal of stitches, together with an indication of the type of suture thread is described in the table 1.

On the face, where the scar will be visible, it is important to remove stitches as soon as possible, while Steri-Strip ® is placed for 7 extra days, since during this period there is risk of wound dehiscence after minor trauma. In other anatomical regions, where the cosmetic result is not as important and the healing process is not as fast as in the face, the sutures should be left longer. In particular, in periarticular areas –due to continuous movement, and in the lower extremities, where the healing process is slower, the stitches will be removed later than usual.

Suturing needles

Needles are designed to carry the suture through tissues with minimal damage. Needle selection depends on the type of tissue to be sutured, its accessibility and suture thickness.

There are straight needles which are handled with the fingers, and are not used in minor surgery, and curved needles, which are handled with the needle holder, allowing greater accuracy and accessibility. Curved needles have different arcs, those of 3 / 8 circle or ½ circle being the most useful in minor surgery.

According to their section, needles are classified as triangular, conical or spatulate. Triangular needles have sharp edges that allow suturing through highly-resistent tissues such as skin, subcutaneous tissue and fascia and, therefore, are considered as first choice in minor surgery.

Curved needles are used with the needle holder, since its jaws are especially designed to hold needles safely and atraumatically. Needle holders should be selected in accordance with the size of the needle and the surgical area (shorter needle holders are preferred in minor surgery).

Staples

staples are available in different widths (W: Wide staples, R: normal staples) and are applied by disposable staplers preloaded with a variable number of staples (35 staples for large staplers, 10 for small ones). The use of staples versus conventional sutures has certain advantages such as the speed with which the suture is performed, low resistance and no tissue reaction

Indications: In linear wounds on the scalp, trunk and limbs, and for temporary closure of wounds in patients to be transferred or with other serious injuries.

Contraindications: Wounds on face and hands. Staple use is contraindicated in regions that are going to be studied through CT or MRI.

Staple application and removal: Staples are applied with the dominant hand, while the nondominant hand everts the skin edges using dissecting forceps with teeth. Time for staple removal parallels time for suture removal in each anatomical region. Staple removal is performed using a staple extractor which is also provided by the stapler distributor.

Adhesive sutures

Adhesive sutures consist of adhesive tapes made of porous paper and capable of approximating the edges of a wound or incision. Sterile presentations are available in various widths and lengths, but can be cut to the proper size as required. Their advantages over conventional sutures are speed and ease of application. Besides, local anesthesia is not necessary and no "suture cross-hatching" is produced.

Indications: linear and superficial wounds with little tension. The regions where they are used most are: the forehead, chin, malar eminence, chest, non-articular surfaces of the limbs and fingertips. They are also a good choice for elderly patients and patients under treatment with corticosteroids, whose skin is thin and fragile and as wound-reinforcement after stitch removal.

Contraindications: irregular wounds, wounds closed under tension, wounds producing continous oozing or discharge, wounds on the scalp and hairy areas, skin folds and joint surfaces

Application and removal of adhesive sutures: The wound should be dry, free of blood or secretions; substances may be added to increase skin adhesiveness. The suture tape is cut, before removing its protective paper, to the adequate size and is then applied to the wound using dissecting forceps without teeth or fingers, first on one edge of the wound and then the other and along the wound.

Time for adhesive suture removal parallels time for conventional suture removal in each anatomical region. Unlike conventional sutures, any wound closed with adhesive suture should not be wet for the first few days, due to the risk of tape detachment.

Tissue adhesives (glues)

One of the latest advances in the treatment of wounds has been the development of tissue adhesives. These products (cyanoacrylates) act as an adhesive, producing an epidermal plane closure, so they are used as topical agents that bind to the most superficial epithelial layer (stratum corneum) and hold together the wound edges. The product forms a bridge over the edges of wounds, lacerations and incisions, holding them together for 7 to 14 days. During this lapse of time, normal wound reparation takes place under the adhesive. After 7 to 14 days, most of the adhesive is shed along with the stratum corneum before degradation occurs.

In the areas of greatest wound tension or in deeper wounds, cyanoacrylates can be used in conjunction with sutures in the subcutaneous plane.

Application technique

After placing the patient in supine position and once cleaning and hemostasis of the wound have been completed, tissue adhesive will be applied as follows:

- Accurately approximate the wound edges using fingers or dissecting forceps.
- Apply the adhesive on the outer surface of the skin, preventing it from entering the interior of the wound.

- Keep the edges in contact for 30 to 60 seconds. After this time a proper degree of polymerization will have been reached. Final adhesive tension is reached within two minutes of application, and can be checked by gently pulling appart the wound edges. The application process is repeated an average of three times. After polymerization the wound can be inspected through the transparent adhesive film.
- After adhesive application, the wound does not require dressings. The wound should be kept dry 5 days and then it can get wet with caution, avoiding prolonged contact with water (bath). The glue will disappear after 7-10 days

Warnings for correct use

Should the adhesive penetrate within a wound, it will be considered a foreing body and will be eliminated through debridement. Should it contact the eyes, use of an ophthalmic ointment is recommended, since its emollients will facilitate the removal of the adhesive, along with ocular occlusion for twenty-four hours. The adhesive is usually easily detached from the eyelashes, without any need for cutting them. Should the adhesive reach the cornea, it can be extracted as a foreign body or a conservative attitude may be adopted, waiting for spontaneous detachment.

Current indications

Tissue adhesives are a good alternative for closing lacerations that meet the following criteria[1,8]:

- Require 4 / 0 or finer sutures
- Not associated with multiple trauma
- In patients without peripheral vascular disease, diabetes mellitus, bleeding diathesis, history of keloid formation
- The cause of the wound is not an animal bite, puncture, presure sore, or crush injury causing stellate lacerations
- Wound should present no visual sign of local or systemic active infection, contamination or visible or devitalized tissue within an active rash
- Not located in lip vermillion, mucous membranes or very hairy areas

4. Surgical procedures and techniques of anesthesia in minor surgery

4.1 Basic surgical maneuvers

Practice of minor surgical procedures requires knowledge of proper technique for handling surgical instruments (described above). Surgical knowledge and technique are also essential for carrying out minor surgical procedures.

The practice of any surgical procedure, however minimal, is not without risks. The possibility of complications during and after surgery must always be kept in mind. A satisfactory outcome of surgery should never be guaranteed, since the results of surgical treatment are not always predictable, and depend on many factors, involving not only the physician's skills, but also the patient.

Surgical incision and dissection

A correct design of the incision is important in any cutting technique, so that enough exposure of the lesion is obtained without damaging any important anatomical structures and, at the same time, a cosmetically acceptable scar is produced. It is therefore essential to know the anatomy of the area being treated, as well as the basic technique for obtaining optimal cosmetic and functional results.

Dissection is a maneuver that involves detaching layers of tissue similar to others to which they are attached. There are two ways to dissect tissue: a so-called blunt dissection (in which tissue is not sectioned but spread apart and is usually performed using Metzembaun scissors or mosquito forceps) and a cutting dissection, which is done with a scalpel or scissors. In minor surgery, the most common level of dissection should be: for the face and neck, the junction between the dermis and subcutaneous tissue, for the scalp, the subgaleal plane, and for the trunk and extremities, the junction between the superficial and deep fascia

Incisions in minor surgery

To plan a surgical incision certain elements, such as the anatomy of the surgical area, the relaxed skin tension lines and the biology of the lesion to be treated must be taken into consideration.

Surgical incisions or excisions should be oriented so that they result in an acceptable scar, both cosmetically and functionally. To do this, incisions must parallel the minimal tension lines, which match facial expression lines and skin relaxation lines (Fig 8). Diagrams of the relaxed skin tension lines are available for correct incision planning.

Design of the incisions or excisions also must take into account the type of lesion to be treated. For excisional biopsies, it is necessary to leave an adequate margin (1-2 mm) of healthy skin both around the lesion and in depth, depending on each lesion. For partial or incisional biopsies, the incision should be designed so that it can be included in a future excision.
In many cases, marking the planned incision helps the surgeon not to lose reference after draping of the surgical field. The incision can be marked prior to skin antiseptic preparation or a previously sterilized marking pen can be used in the surgical field after skin preparation and draping.

Types of incisions for minor surgery

Incision: Used for surgical exposure of deeper tissues (e.g., lipomas, epidermal cysts, lymph node biopsies) or for drainage of abscesses. Incisions can be straight, angled or curved depending on the anatomic area involved and the type of surgery.

Elliptical excision: Used to remove skin lesions with a margin of healthy skin around the lesion and in depth. As a general rule, the length of the ellipse should be 3 times its width and the ends must form a 30- degree angle (Fig 9). It should be oriented along the lines of minimal tension and not along the axis of the lesion to be excised.

Tangential Excision: Also called "skin shave", it involves the removal by scalpel or scissors of very superficial lesions, eliminating only the most superficial layers of the skin. The defect created is allowed to heal by secondary intention. Shave can only be used to remove certain lesions affecting only the most superficial layers of the skin and for which diagnosis is certain.

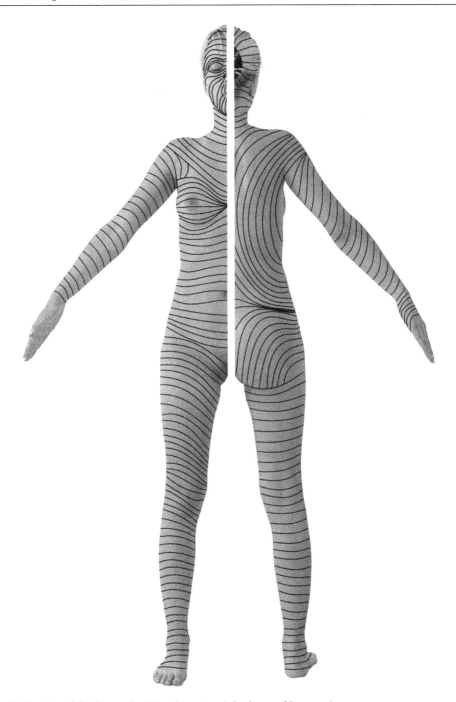

Fig. 8. Graphs of the lines of minimal tension (the lines of Langers)

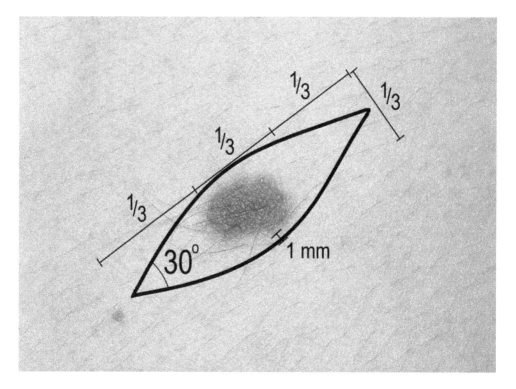

Fig. 9. Characteristics of the Elliptical excision.

Haemostasis

It is a surgical maneuver that not only controls bleeding, but allows clear vision of surgical anatomy. Most episodes of bleeding in minor surgery (where incisions or injuries very rarely involve major blood vessels) are controllable with pressure with a gauze or surgical towel. Moreover, applying a compressive bandage on the wound in the immediate postoperative period reduces the possibility of collecting a hematoma or seroma.

Types of hemostasis

- A *tourniquet* is not a method of hemostasis "per se", but provides temporary control of bleeding, allowing wound exploration and reducing surgical time. Its use in minor surgery is limited to the fingers (nail surgery, etc) and should not exceed 15 minutes.
- *Hemostats.* After identifying a bleeding vessel, the surgeon clampes it with the tip of a toothless-hemostat and checks the interruption of bleeding. Attempts to clamp blindly a bleeding vessel in the depth of a bleeding wound must be avoided at all costs because of the risk of damaging important structures (eg nerves or tendons).
- *Ligatures* are threads that, when tied around a blood vessel, occlude its lumen and prevent bleeding. After identification of the bleeding vessel, it should be fixed using a hemostat. The ligature (a single 3/0 thread) should be passed below the clamp and several knots tied. The ends are left short.

- In hemostasis by *electrocoagulation* the bovie is used in coagulation mode.

Suture techniques

Their goal is to approximate similar tissues so that proper healing of the wound ensues. For an optimal surgical closure the following principles should be remembered:

1. Tension must be avoided: suturing a wound under tension decreases the blood supply to its edges, increasing healing problems and the risk of infection.

2. Eversion of the wound edges: due to the tendency of scars to contract over time, if surgical edges are left slightly elevated above the plane of the skin, they will flatten over time, producing a more cosmetically acceptable result. One of the keys to proper surgical skin edge eversion is to introduce the needle at a 90-degree angle with the plane of the skin so that the suture, once tied, lifts the skin (fig 10).

3. Closure by layers: for most minor surgical interventions a single (cutaneous) layer closure is enough. However, if there is any tension, if the wound is very deep and involves several surgical layers or if there is much dead space, a multi-layer closure may become necessary. A multi-layer wound closure requires thick fascia or dermis for the placement of internal sutures, because fatty tissue lacks consistency to support sutures.

4. Type of suture material: it is a less important factor than the previous principles. If a suture is removed too late it will cause scarring in the areas of entry and exit of the suture ("cross-hatching"). To avoid it, stitches shall be removed as soon points as possible. The choice of suture material and its thickness are also important.

Interrupted sutures

Interrupted sutures are those in which each stitch is independent of the next one. Interrupted suturing is the most appropriate suturing technique for minor surgery, as it helps to distribute stress, promotes the drainage of the wound and stitch removal is easier.

Simple stitch (percutaneous): it is the suture technique of choice for skin suturing in minor procedures and is used alone or in combination with buried stitches in deeper wounds.

Simple stitch with inverted knot (buried): Used to approximate the deep planes, reducing tension, and to obliterate dead spaces before skin suturing. It is not necessary in superficial wounds. Absorbable material is used, leaving the knot in the depth of the wound, thus reducing the chances of suture exposure through the incision. The knot is cut flush to decrease the amount of foreign material within the wound.

Mattress stitch or "U" stitch: vertical mattress stitch: a stitch useful in areas of loose skin (back of the hand, elbow), where the wound edges tend to invaginate. In addition to providing good eversion of wound edges, this suture provides good obliteration of dead space, avoiding the need for buried sutures in shallow wounds.

Horizontal mattress stitch: This stitch also provides a good eversion of wound edges, especially in areas where the dermis is thick (e.g. Palm of the hand and sole of the foot).

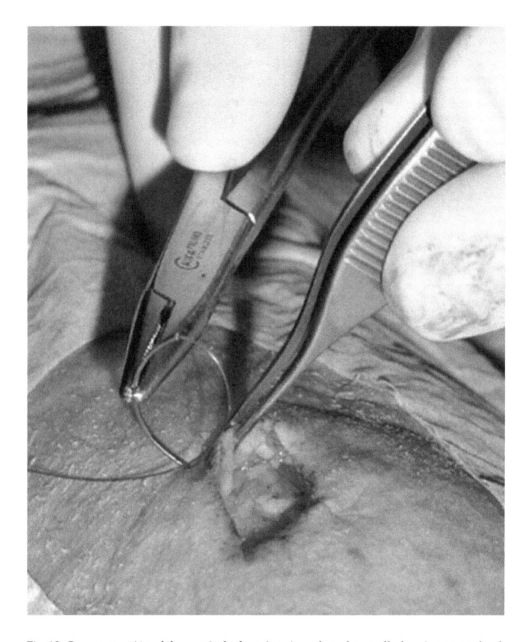

Fig. 10. Correct eversión of the surgical edges, is to introduce the needle forming an angle of 90 ° with the plane of the skin

Half-buried horizontal mattress stitch: is used to suture wound angles or surgical edges of uneven thickness.

Running sutures

They impede the drainage of the wound, so they are contraindicated if infection is suspected and in heavily contaminated wounds. Suture removal is somewhat more difficult, and there is no chance to remove stitches in several sessions.

Simple running suture: It is a sequence of stitches with an initial and a final knot. It takes short time to perform but it makes difficult to adjust skin tension and does not always provide adequate wound edge eversion. It is seldom used in minor surgery.

Intradermal (subcuticular) running suture: This type of suture allows wound suturing without breaking the skin, prevents "cross-hatching" and provides an optimal cosmetic result. It is performed by passing the suture through the dermis horizontally along the entire wound. At both ends suture can go out through the skin (removable intradermal suture), for which nonabsorbable monofilament suture material is selected or a knot may be tied inside the wound (non- removable intradermal suture) for which absorbable material is used. Use of multifilament suture material as silk for intradermal suturing should be avoided, as it would be very difficult to remove the suture material. Intradermal sutures are used on wounds where it will be necessary to maintain the suture a long time (more than 15 days). There should be no tension on the wound. In minor surgery their usefulness is limited.

Knot-tying

Instrumental knot-tying is performed with a needle holder and a curved needle. In minor surgery, where the surgical area is superficial and accessible to surgical instruments, *instrumental knot-tying* is the preferred technique because it provides more precise suturing and significant savings in suture material, except for suture-ligation of small blood vessels, where *manual tying* is preferred. The recommended technique is the surgeon's knot which consists of a double loop followed by several simple loops. The advantage of this knot is the resistance of its first double loop, which prevents knot untying as the surgeon proceeds with the following loops.

When knot-tying a multifilament thread (e.g. Silk) three loops are usually enough (first a double loop plus two single loops). When knot-tying a monofilament thread (eg. Nylon, polypropylene) an extra loop should be added, to increase knot security.

The knots should be placed to one side of the wound, instead of placing them on top of the incision. This will allow better visualization of the wound, interfere less with the healing and facilitate stitch removal.

4.2 Techniques of local anesthesia in minor surgery

Local anesthetics are drugs that block the transmission of nerve impulses causing, at least, the absence of pain sensation in the area of injection.

According to a small chemical difference, local anesthetics can be classified into two groups:

Esters (procaine, tetracaine, chloroprocaine, benzocaine.... which is obsolete due to its high incidence of sensitization) and amides (lidocaine, mepivacaine, bupivacaine, prilocaine, etidocaine and ropivacaine). For their remarkable safety and efficacy we will .only use amides, namely lidocaine and mepivacaine

Available presentations

The concentration of the anesthetic is expressed in%. We must know that a concentration of 1% means that 100 ml of the solution contain 1 g of anesthetic and 10 ml of the solution contain 100 mg of the anesthetic. To calculate the concentration in mg / ml, the concentration percent should be multiplied by 10; thus, a 2 ml ampoule of 2% mepivacaine contains 20 mg of mepivacaine for each ml of the solution, i.e. this 2 ml ampoule contain 40 mg of mepivacaine.

Maximum doses and features

LIDOCAINE.- 10 ml Amp. ◊ 1% (100 mg), 2% (200 mg), 5% (500 mg)
Dose without vasoconstrictor: 3-4 mg / kg ◊ maximum 300 mg (3 amp 10 ml 1%)
Dose with vasoconstrictor: 7 mg / kg ◊ maximum 500 mg (5 amp 10 ml 1%)
Onset of action: 2-4 min. Induces vasodilation.
Duration: 1-2 hours, depending on the dose and breadth of the area.

In adults, concentration should range between 0.5 and 1% and total dose should not exceed 30 ml.

In children, concentration should range between 0.25 and 0.50% and total dose should not exceed 4 mg / kg.

MEPIVACAINE.- 10 ml Amp. 1% (100 mg) and 2 ml Amp. 2% (40 mg)
Dose without vasoconstrictor: 400 mg (4-5 mg / kg)
Dose with vasoconstrictor. 500mg (7mg/Kg)
Onset of action: 2-5 min. Induces less vasodilation.
Duration: 1-1.5 hours, depending on the dose and breadth of the area.

In adults, mepivacaine should be used at a 1% concentration and total dose should not exceed 40 ml.

For children 0.25 to 0.50% mepivacaine should be used and total dose should not exceed 7 mg / kg.

Adverse effects of local anesthetics

- *Local effects*: Pain, hematoma, injury to nerve trunks.
- *Systemic effects*: 1. Due to overdose toxicity. These effects appear when the maximum recommended dose is exceeded or the correct dosage is used but applied intravascularly. From a clinical standpoint, toxicity is associated to the central nervous system (CNS: tinnitus, metallic taste, numbness, dizziness, twitching, etc.) and cardiovascular system (CV: hypotension, arrhythmias, cardiac arrest). 2. Due from an allergic reaction. 3. Due to psychogenic reaction (vasovagal syncope), this is the most common adeverse effect.

Use of vasoconstrictors

The asociation of vasoconstrictors with local anesthetics improves the safety profile of the anesthetic and also allows for better visualization of the surgical field. The most widely used is adrenaline and the maximum dose (as a vasoconstrictor) must not exceed 250 micrograms in adults or 10 micrograms / kg in children.

The recommended concentration is a dilution of 1:100,000 or 1:200,000 (best) which is prepared by mixing 0.1 mg of adrenaline (0.1 ml of 1:1000 adrenaline) in 10 ml of anesthetic to obtain a 1:100,000 dilution, or in 20 ml to obtain a 1:200,000 dilution.

Due to the risk of necrosis and delayed healing, adrenaline should not be used in acral areas (fingers and toes,), or in devitalized or traumatized skin. Except in such circumstances, using the anesthetic with vasoconstrictor is highly recommended.

Basic techniques of local anesthesia

Topical anesthesia

In recent years, topical anesthetics have been developed as an alternative to infiltration both for intact skin and for lacerations and mucosae, especially in children. Topical anesthetics used in minor surgical procedures and their characteristics are shown in the table 2:

Anesthetic	Mode of use	characteristics	Indications	Complications	Not indicated
LET® (4 % lidocaine, 0,1 % epinephine 1:2000, 0,5 % tetracaíne)	1-3 ml applied directly on wound for 15-30 min	Onset 20-30 min after aplication. Duration of effect has not been clearly established	Can be effective in children for face and scalp lacerations and less effective in limbs	No important adverse effects reported	For mucosae and acral areas
EMLA® lidocaine 25 mg/ml plus prilocaine 25 mg/ml,	1-2 gr of cream should be applied for each 10 cm2 of intact skin and occluded Or apply in patch Maximum dose is 10 grams	Onset 60-120 min after aplication. Duration of effect is 30-120 min. not useful on palms of hands and soles of feet	Admitted for procedures on intact skin: scraping and shaving (seborrheic keratosis, Molluscum contagiosum, dermal nevus), cryosurgery (warts, condylomas), electrosurgery (small fibroids and spiders), laser hair removal, pre-anesthesia for infiltration	Local mild irritation, contact dermatitis. There have been reports of Metahemoglo binemia in children aged <6 months	For wounds or deep tissues

Table 2. Topical anesthetics used in minor surgical procedures and their characteristics

Infiltration anesthesia: angular and peri-lesional[9]

1. *Angular infiltration*: From the point of entry, the anesthetic is infiltrated in three or more different directions, like a fan (Fig 11).
2. *Perilesional infiltration*: Starting from each point of entry the anesthetic is infiltrated in a single direction, so that after several injections, the lesion will have been surrounded by anesthetic, and the diferent points of entry will be forming a polyhedral figure (Fig 12).
3. *Linear Infiltration*: If the lesion to be operated on is a skin laceration, the anesthetic should be directly infiltrated into the wound edges in a linear fashion. If the wound is

bruised and has irregular edges, it is preferable to use a perilesional technique from the uninjured area, and follow along the margins of the wound to avoid introducing microbial contamination.

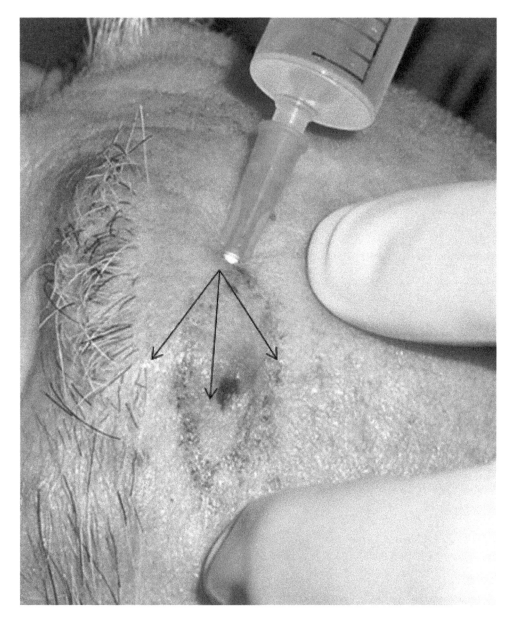

Fig. 11. Anesthesic angular infiltration: it infiltrates following three or more different directions, like a fan

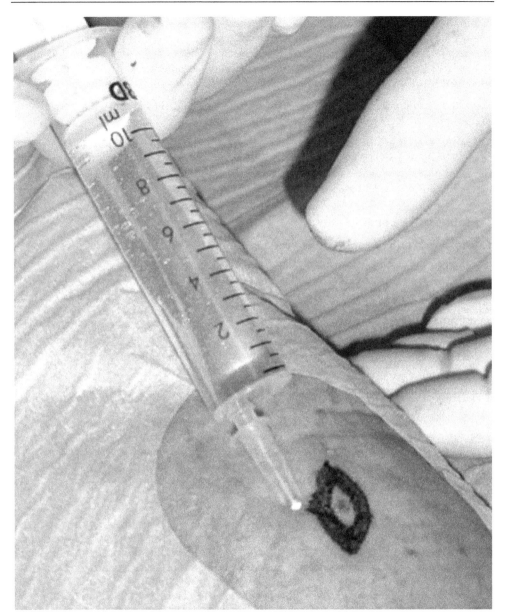

Fig. 12. Infiltration perilesional: the injury surrounds itself by means of different infiltrations

Loco-regional block

There are multiple blocks, digital blocks being the most common minor surgery. The digital block will allow the surgeon to act on all types of fingers injuries (lacerations, wound debridement, soft tissue injuries, foreign body removal, pathology of the nail).

A thin needle is inserted at the base of the proximal phalanx in a dorsal and lateral location. The needle is inserted to the point where the collateral palmar digital nerve should lie and, after aspiration, 0.5-1 mL of local anesthetic is injected. The needle is removed until its tip is just below the skin and, after aspiration, a dose of anesthetic is again infiltrated in a subcutaneous plane along the side of the base of the phalanx.

Then, the needle will be inserted on the opposite side and infiltration will proceed in a similar way.

Before the procedure, the surgeon should wait 10-15 minutes for a complete effect of the block. The total injected volume should not exceed 4 ml, because higher volumes can compress digital vessels and cause ischemia. For the same reason, anesthetics used in digital blocks should contain no vasoconstrictor.

5. Preoperative considerations

5.1 Diagnostic criteria for the most common lesions in minor surgery

The indications for minor surgery are related to the diagnosis of the patient's lesion. A misdiagnosis can cause incorrect treatment and lead to loss of clinical information relevant to the patient's prognosis. It is therefore imperative that general practitioners have an extensive knowledge of the lesions most frequently treated by minor surgery. When in doubt about the nature of any given lesion, preoperative diagnosis should always be confirmed by other specialists[10]. For each lesion there is a surgical procedure of choice. Other techniques may also be valid or they may even be contraindicated.

The following paragraphs contain an overview of the most important diagnostic consideration in lesions usually treated with minor surgery.

Seborrheic keratoses

Seborrheic keratoses are benign light brown lesions initially measuring 1-3 mm which after years of growth can turn into more or less pigmented 1-6 cm plaques with a rough or waxy surface. These lesions are easily treated with curettage, electrosurgery or cryosurgery. In case of doubt, an incisional biopsy should be sent for histopathological analysis.

Epidermal cysts

Also known as epithelial cysts, epidermoid cysts or sebaceous cysts, they are firm nodules, measuring from 0.2 to 5 cm in diameter, formed by a layer of stratified squamous epithelium or epithelium of a hair follicle, which are located in the dermis or subcutaneous tissue. They are not adherent to deep tissues and in many instances a central keratin- rich pore can be seen. Queratin is the main component inside the cyst. The most common location is on the face, neck, chest, upper third of back and scrotum. Their treatment is surgical removal for cosmetic reasons or due to recurrent infections

Warts

They are a form of benign epithelial hyperplasia induced by human papilloma virus (HPV). The clinical presentations of the cutaneous infection by HPV include:

Verruca Vulgaris: The treatment of choice is 15-20% salicylic acid with petroleum jelly, applied topically for 2-3 weeks or liquid nitrogen.

Plantar wart: The treatment of choice is 40% salicylic acid with petroleum jelly, applied topically for 3 weeks followed first by curettage and then by liquid nitrogen. Surgery and electrocoagulation are not indicated

Molluscum

Pearly white papules of 1-5 mm (sometimes even bigger) with central dimpling. They may appear isolated or in groups in the neck, trunk, anogenital area or eyelids. They are very common in children and in patients with HIV / AIDS with extensive lesions which difficult to eradicate.

Their first choice treatment is cryosurgery, curettage or electrodesiccation.

Lipoma

Lipomas are slow-growing benign tumors of mature adipose tissue. They are a frequent cause of consultation due to mechanical or aesthetic reasons. Lipomas appear as soft, elastic, smooth or multilobulated tumors of variable size (from 1 or 2 cm to 15 cm or more) with ill-defined borders, and not adherent to deep planes.

Lipomas are generally asymptomatic and patients usually refer the emergence of a "lump" whose location, size and visibility will determine how urgent such consultation will be. In most cases, a simple physical examination will establish a correct diagnosis of lipoma.

Lipomas are treated by surgical removal. Their removal by either a general practitioner or a surgeon usually depends on the size, location and positionof the lipoma in the subcutaneous plane.

Fibroma pendulum, skin tags

These are pedunculated fleshy-looking benign tumours, whose colour is either similar to that of the surrounding skin or darker. Their size varies from a few mm (which usually appear in groups and are located in the neck, armpits, and skin folds) up to 2-5 mm (which usually appear as pedunculated and solitary lesions).

Their treatment is justified for cosmetic reasons, and good surgical results usually ensue. These lesions can be treated by skin shave, electrodesiccation and cryosurgery.

Melanocytic nevi

They are acquired lesions in the form of macules or papules or small nodules (<1 cm) and are constituted by groups of melanocytes located in the epidermis, dermis or both areas and rarely in the subcutaneous tissue. They are very common in Caucasians and family incidence has been clearly established. Sun exposure contributes to the induction of these lesions.

Most appear in early childhood and peak in young adults to regress and disappear gradually and are asymptomatic. By contrast, dysplastic nevi continue to appear as new lesions over a lifetime and do not show signs of involution. The indication for removal will be established when any of the following characteristics is seen:

- Presentation site: scalp, mucous membranes, anogenital area
- Time of evolution: de novo appearance in adulthood
- Color: variegated or modified
- Borders: always have been irregular or have just turned irregular

- Symptoms: If the nevus starts to itch, bleed or hurt
- Epiluminescence microscopy: criteria of dysplasia

Actinic keratoses

These are yellowish brown dry- looking maculopapular lesions, with a rough and scaly texture located in sun-exposed areas of middle-aged patients. Actinic keratoses are more prevalent in males. Most of these lesions are present on the skin for years and 13-25% of them will lead to a squamous cell carcinoma.

The treatment of choice is the topical application of 5% 5-fluorouracil or Imiquimod. If lesions are scarce and localized, they may be treated with liquid nitrogen.

Basal cell carcinoma

Basal cell carcinoma is the most common skin malignancy. Although it can occur at any age, its incidence raises abruptly after the age of 40 with a history of heavy sun exposure. These lesions are more prevalent in the face and scalp followed by the ears and upper chest and back.

Excision should be considered for any slow-growing pale pink, brown or flesh-colored, flat or slightly elevated new skin lesion located in the face, ear, neck, back or scalp with a pearly or waxy appearance, that also meets any of the following criteria:

- Blood vessels visible in the lesion or in the adjacent skin
- Keratin pearls sometimes visible with a loupe
- Appearance of a scar with no history of previous wound in the area
- Non-healing ulcer

Squamous cell Carcinoma

This is a malignant tumor that usually appears on a previous premalignant lesion.

It takes different clinical forms, in this case as a crust-covered superficial ulcer that grows insidiously over months. In other cases it may appear as a hard papule or nodule.

Squamous-cell carcinomas require a multidisciplinary therapeutical approach involving dermatologists, surgeons, radiotherapists, and chemotherapists.

Melanoma

Of all skin malignancies, melanoma has the worst prognosis. There are different clinical presentations and, for their detection, the "ABCDE-rule of melanoma" , which is described in the following table, should never be overlooked (Table 3).

	A-B-C-D-E rule for any lesion clinically suspicious of melanoma
A	Asimetry
B	Border: irregular and scalloped
C	Colour: mottled, irregular shades of brown, black, gray and pink
D	Diameter over 6 mm
E	Subtle or obvious skin elevation (on illuminated sideview) and serial assessment of growth

Table 3. A-B-C-D-E rule for any lesion clinically suspicious of melanoma

Any lesion suspicious of melanoma should be referred to a dermatologist. These lesions should never undergo biopsy by skin shave or curettage, nor should any destructive procedure (cryosurgery or electrosurgery) be used in their diagnosis or therapy.

5.2 Body areas of risk in minor surgery

Certain body areas are considered high-risk areas for minor surgical procedures, due to the superficial location of some anatomical structures, which are likely to be injured during surgery. To avoid injury to these structures, it is necessary to know their theoretical path and keep the surgery, whenever possible, on a superficial plane (superficial subcutaneous tissue). Other areas are also considered high-risk areas due to the potential esthetic impact of poor surgical technique.

High-risk areas for minor surgery include the facial and cervical regions, axillary and supraclavicular regions, wrists, hands and fingers, the groin, the popliteal fossa and the feet (Fig 13 A, B).

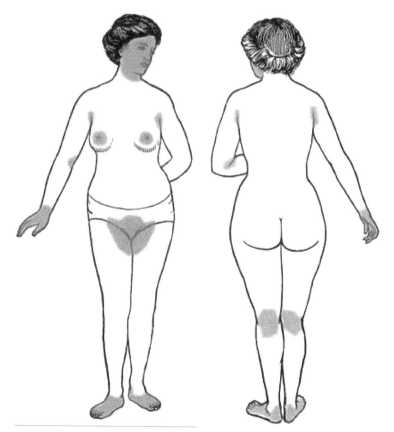

Fig. 13, A, B: The zones of risk in Minor Surgery include the facial and cervical region, the region axilar and supraclavicular, the wrists, hands and fingers, the inguinal region, the hollow poplíteo and the feet

Along with the previously-mentioned areas, we must also consider those regions with a greater tendency to develop pathological scars. The deltoid and shoulder region, the sternal and interscapular region, and the skin of black patients and children are especially prone to hypertrophic scarring and keloids. Thus, before any skin lesion is removed in any of these areas it is important to discuss this possibility with the patient, especially in cases where the excision pursues aesthetic improvent, and is not indicated for diagnostic or therapeutic reasons.

6. How to perform a surgical procedure: Elliptical excision step by step

Elliptical excision is a skin excision technique with a spindle-shaped design. This ellipse should include all skin layers plus some subcutaneous fat, in order to remove skin lesions with a safety margin both around and under them. This technique not only allows for simultaneous diagnosis and treatment, but also facilitates closure producing good cosmetic results. It is, therefore, the ideal technique to remove the majority of skin lesions[11-14].

Before surgery the patient should be informed about the procedure and its technical details before asking them to sign the informed consent form.

The procedure involves the following steps:

1. **Design of the incision** which is drawn with a marker using the following parameters: the longitudinal axis of the ellipse will be three times longer than its transverse axis and will be parallel to skin tension lines. Its ends will form a <30 °angle to avoid "dog ears". There must be a 1-2 mm margin between the lesion and the incision (some lesions may require more generous margins).
2. **Preparation of the surgical field**: cleaning and antisepsis
3. **Local anesthetic** injection, covering the entire edge of the incision and the tissue to be sectioned and sutured
4. **Superficial skin incision** along the marked ellipse, going through the entire dermis to prevent jagged edges. The incision is made with a clean cut of the scalpel, which is held like a pencil, and any sawing movement should be avoided. Using the nondominant hand, the skin should be stretched or pinched along the previously marked incision line (Fig 14).
5. **En bloc excision of the lesion** using the nondominant hand the skin is stretched with toothed-forceps from one end of the ellipse and, using the edge of the blade, the deep wedge-shaped incision is made (always under direct vision, Fig 15), until fat is reached and the lesion is, thus, removed en bloc.
6. **Haemostasis of the surgical area**: if anesthesia with vasoconstrictor is used bleeding will be scarce and hemostasis will be easily achieved by applying digital pressure with a gauze.
7. **Wound closure** by layers: most minor surgical procedures only require suturing of the skin surface, but if there is any tension, the incision is deep and involves several tissue layers or there is dead space, suturing several surgical planes may be required. The deep-layer suture should be performed with absorbable material using an inverted-knot technique. Then, the superficial closure with nonabsorbable suture will be performed. The number of stitches will depend on the tension of the wound, suture thickness and chosen suture technique (Fig 16).
8. **Sterile dressing** placement after cleaning the surgical área

9. **Submission of the resected specimen to pathology**, in a container with 10% formalin.
10. **Follow-up**: After 48 hours the wound can be washed gently, and the patient should be warned of postoperative risks and taught how to take care of the surgical wound. No surgical procedure is complete until the pathology report has been received and the patient informed of the results and prognosis.

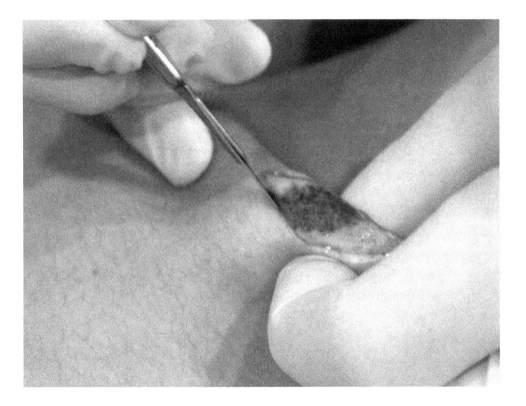

Fig. 14. Incision is done giving a clean cut of the scalpel, not sawing, taking the handle of the scalpel as a pencil, traccionando (or pinching the zone) with the fingers

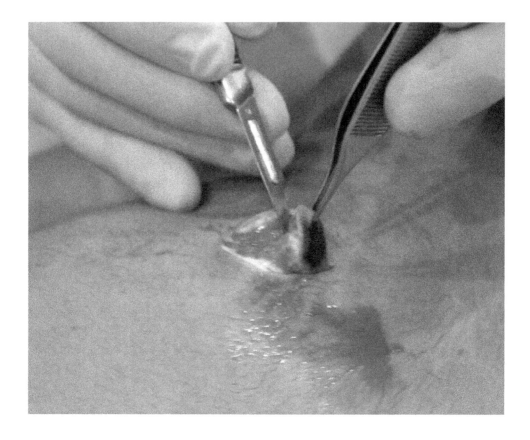

Fig. 15. En bloc excision: traction is realized (with forceps with teeth) from an end of the spindle and with the edge of the scalpel deep incision is realized

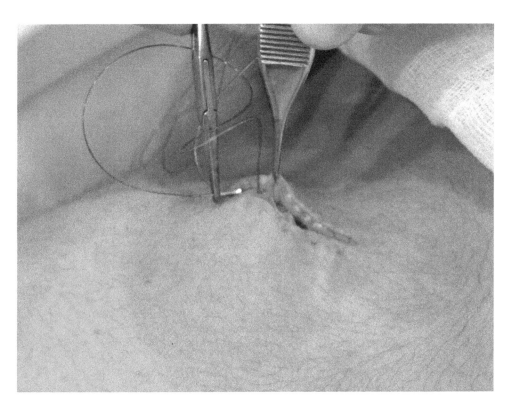

Fig. 16. Suturing of the skin surface

7. Good clinical practice in minor surgery

Preoperative

For most basic minor surgical procedures, no preoperative work-up is needed. However, since we, as general practitioners, operate on our own patients, we have inmediate access to their medical history which can completed with a series of simple questions that will help us detect those patients in whom surgery poses especial risks or is contraindicated. The table 4 summarizes the precautions of minor surgery in primary care:

- Diabetes Mellitus and peripheral vascular diseasse when planning surgery in the lower extremities

- In patients with chronic use of immunosuppressors (corticosteroids)

- Do not add vasoconstrictor to local anesthetic in patients with: arrhythmia, severe hypertension, hyperthyroidism, pheochromocytoma, pregnancy, and in anesthesia of the fingers

- Anatomic areas of risk

- Use of oral anticoagulants and antiplatelet agents should be sought for. The risk-benefit of their suspension should be studied prior to surgery.
In most patients at low risk, minor surgical procedures can be performed without altering the anticoagulation regimen if their INR is within therapeutic range (*Antithrombotic and Thrombolytic Therapy: American College of Chest Physicians Evidence-Based Clincial Practice Guidelines (8th Edition)2008*)

Specific precautions with the use of electrocautery
- Keep the patient's skin clear from any metallic object. Metal dentures, implants, prosthesis, IUD are not contraindicated
- Do not use alcohol or use the bovie near a source of oxygen.
- Use latex gloves for insulation

Special precautions for cryosurgery
- Patients with areas of potential circulatory compromise due to the risk of necrosis.
- Hairy areas in which hair loss could ensue.
- Hyperpigmented areas (black or dark skin), where the use of cryosurgery can leave areas of hypopigmentation.
- Patients with high levels of cryoglobulins.

Table 4. Precautions minor surgery

Premedication

In patients with increased anxiety, use of preoperative sedation can be considered. 5-10 mg oral or sublingual diazepam, or 1-5 mg sublingual lorazepam can be administered 30 minutes before surgery.

Contraindications for minor surgery

- With few justified exceptions, no malignant skin lesion should be surgically treated by the general practitioner. Similarly, all lesions labeled as malignant after pathological analysis, should promt consultation with other specialists.
- Allergy to local anesthetics: If there is doubt about a history of allergic reactions, the patient should see the allergist prior to surgery.
- Pregnancy: If the patient is pregnant, surgery should be deferred until the end of pregnancy, to avoid unnecessary risks. If malignancy is suspected, the patient should be referred to a specialist.

- Acute intercurrent disease: if the patient suffers an acute illness at the time of surgery (heart failure, liver failure, arrhythmia, flu or pneumonia), surgery should be postponed until recovery.
- Doubt about patient's motivations: surgery is contraindicated in patients whose motivation is questionable or in whom there is excessive preoccupation about the aesthetic result
- Patients with psychiatric disorders or uncooperative patients are not eligible for surgery in primary care. In general it is not advisable to involve uncooperative patients.
- Refusal to sign the informed consent form is a contraindication for any minor surgery procedure or technique.

Intraoperative complications

Vasovagal syncope is the most fequent complication and is more common in young men. Warning signs are flushing, pallor, sweating, weakness, nausea (occasionally, vomiting), etc. After these simptoms, some patients may lose consciousness.

Treatment consists of placing the patient in Trendelenburg's position, administering oxygen and i.v. fluids if needed and, in severe cases (long-lasting or associated with bradycardia) use of 0.5-1 mg sc or iv atropine can be considered (maximum dose, 2 mg). Generally, most of patients recover spontaneously over a period of seconds to a few minutes.

All medical premises where minor surgical procedures are performed should have CPR equipment and medication.

Postoperative complications

- Hematoma-seroma: fluid collection under the sutures that occurs whenever cavities or dead space have been left in the surgical site. To prevent their formation, a correct intraoperative hemostasis is paramount plus suturing the wound in layers with no gaps and, finally, applying a compressive bandage.
- Infection can occur in up to 1% of minor surgical patients and it appears as swelling, redness of the wound edges and, sometimes, purulent discharge. Symptoms such as fever and / or chills are only rarely seen. Infections are treated by removing some of the stitches, plus daily cleaning and disinfection of the wound and allowing the wound to close by secondary intention. If necessary, a drain may be inserted into the wound and an oral antibiotic regimen may be initiated.
- Wound dehiscence: The separation of the edges of the wound before proper healing. There are predisposing factors secondary to surgery (excessive tension on the edges of the wound, use of inappropriate suture material or early suture withdrawal) or it may be the final phase of other complications such as hematoma or infection. After wound dehiscence, wound repair will take place by secondary intention, resulting in a poor cosmetic result.
- Hypertrophic scar and keloid scarring are deviations from normal wound-repair process. Hypertrophic scars do not grow beyond the initial limits of the primary wound whereas in a keloid the scar tissue extends beyond the initial boundaries of the scar, forming a permanent bulk of scar tissue. Keloids are very difficult to prevent and their most frequent location is in the chest, shoulders and upper back, in young people and

blacks. Treatment of these scars is difficult and results are often discouraging. Occlusive treatment or steroid injections may be tried.

8. References

[1] Arribas JM (2006). Cirugía menor y procedimientos en medicina de familia (2ª edición). Madrid: Jarpyo Editores,

[2] Czarnowski C, Ponka D, Rughani R, Geoffrion P. See one. Do one. Teach one.: Office-based minor surgical procedures. Can Fam Physician. 2008 Jun;54(6):893.

[3] Zuber TJ. Punch biopsy of the skin. Am Fam Physician. 2002 Mar 15;65(6):1155-8, 1161-2, 1164.

[4] Freiman A, Bouganim N. History of cryotherapy. Dermatol Online J. Aug 1 2005;11(2):9

[5] Hainer BL. Electrosurgery for the skin. Am Fam Physician. 2002 Oct 1;66(7):1259-66.

[6] Kudur MH, Pai SB, Sripathi H, Prabhu S. Sutures and suturing techniques in skin closure. Indian J Dermatol Venereol Leprol. 2009 Jul-Aug;75(4):425-34.

[7] Moy RL, Lee A, Zalka A. Commonly used suturing techniques in skin surgery. Am Fam Physician. 1991 Nov;44(5):1625-34.

[8] Singer AJ, Quinn JV, Hollander JE. The cyanoacrylate topical skin adhesives. Am J Emerg Med. 2008 May;26(4):490-6.

[9] Achar S, Kundu S Principles of office anesthesia: part I. Infiltrative anesthesia. Am Fam Physician. 2002 Jul 1;66(1):91-4.

[10] Klaus Wolff y Richard Allen Johnson (2009). Fitzpatrick's Color Atlas and Synopsis of Clinical Dermatology 6th edition. El McGraw-Hill Companies, Inc. New York

[11] Hussain W, Mortimer NJ, Salmon PJ. Optimizing technique in elliptical excisional surgery: some pearls for practice. Br J Dermatol. 2009 Sep;161(3):697-8. Epub 2009 Jun 25.

[12] Czarnowski C, Ponka D, Rughani R, Geoffrion P. Elliptical excision: minor surgery video series. Can Fam Physician. 2008 Aug;54(8):1144

[13] Zuber TJ. Fusiform excision. Am Fam Physician. 2003 Apr 1;67(7):1539-44, 1547-8, 1550.

[14] Wu T. Plastic surgery made easy - simple techniques for closing skin defects and improving cosmetic results. Aust Fam Physician. 2006 Jul;35(7):492-6.

10

Exposure to Environmental Tobacco Smoke in Babies

Lourdes Rofes Ponce[1], Ricardo Almon[2], Elisa Puigdomènech[3],
Manuel A Gomez-Marcos[4] and Carlos Martín-Cantera[5]
[1]Drug Dependency Unit at Sant Joan de Reus Hospital, Reus,
[2]Family Medicine Research Centre School of Health and Medical Sciences,
Örebro University, Örebro,
[3]Lifestyles Research Group from the Primary Health Care Research Unit of Barcelona,
IDIAP Jordi Gol, Barcelona,
[4]Department of Medicine, University of Salamanca,
Cardiovascular Research Group (RETICS RD06/0018/0027, REDIAPP)
Carlos III Institute of Health of the Spanish Ministry of Health,
SACYL, Primary Care Research Unit, La Alamedilla Health Center, Salamanca,
[5]Lifestyles Research Group from the Primary Health Care Research Unit of Barcelona,
IDIAP Jordi Gol, Lifestyles Research Group (RETICS RD06/0018/0027, REDIAPP)
Carlos III Institute of Health of the Spanish Ministry of Health,
Department of Medicine, University Autonomus of Barcelona,
Passeig de Sant Joan Health Center, Barcelona,
[1,3,4,5]Spain
[2]Sweden

1. Introduction

1.1 What is passive smoking?

Passive smoking is defined as the involuntary inhalation of tobacco smoke in closed spaces. It is also known as second hand smoke (SHS) or environmental tobacco smoke (ETS) (ENHS, 2009). ETS includes:

- *Mainstream*: Smoke exhaled by smokers
- *Sidestream*: Smoke produced during the combustion of cigarettes. Approximately 70% of ETS is made by side stream. This smoke is generated by components that escape through every pore of the filter and the paper of the cigarette. The sidestream contains small gaseous particles that can reach peripheral areas of the lung. The sidestream shows 3 more times tar and nicotine than the smoke directly inhaled by the smoker, and 5 more times carbon monoxide (CO) (US Surgeon General, 2006).

In each cigarette, 4000 chemical agents have been found, 43 of them highly toxic such as arsenic, ammonia, benzene, cadmium, hydrogen cyanide, polonium 210, butane, CO, cyanide and acetone (Us Surgeon General, 1989) (see Appendix 1).

Scientific research has demonstrated that pollution caused by tobacco smoke at home can generate higher contamination rates than contamination by industrial air pollution. A series of publications have shown that children are exposed to ETS by 59.4 % - 75 % because of maternal smoking. Up to 70 % of the western children live in houses where at least one of the parents smokes. Thirty percent of these children are exposed to tobacco smoke every day (King et al., 2009).

Passive smoking is the leading cause of preventable death in infancy in industrialized countries (third cause of preventable death in adults), and one of the first leading causes of cancer in developing countries (Seong et al., 2010; Royal College of Physicians, 2010). Some authors estimate that, in Spain, between 1,228-3,237 deaths of lung cancer and cardiovascular diseases are attributable to ETS exposure at home and at work. This circumstances clearly show that exposure to passive smoking is an important public health issue (Lopez et al., 2002).

In 1950 Doll and Hill were the first to publish scientific work related to the harmful health effects of tobacco consumption (Doll & Hill, 1950). In 1974 medical research began to headline harmful effects of ETS on children's health caused by parental smoking (Harlap & Davies, 1974). Furthermore, during the last two decades, international research has found that children of smokers are more likely to be adolescent smokers, probably as a result of role models or easy access to cigarettes (Roseby et al., 2003). Nowadays numerous harmful effects of ETS have been associated with child health (Us Surgeon General, 2006). According to the International Agency for the Research on Cancer (IARC) of the World Health Organization (WHO), ETS is a type A carcinogen and no safety threshold has been established yet (IARC, 2002). Pediatric illnesses and disease related to environmental tobacco smoke are: increased risk of sudden infant death syndrome (SIDS), acute respiratory diseases, respiratory symptoms, aggravation of symptoms in patients with asthma, acute and chronic diseases in the middle ear and slowed lung growth (IARC, 2020; Samet & Sockrider, 2011).

2. Effects of passive smoking in children

2.1 Sudden Infant Death Syndrome (SIDS)

Sudden infant death syndrome (SIDS) can be defined as the sudden and not expected and unexplained death of an infant younger than one year, after a meticulous investigation of potential factors that might have lead to infant death –including an autopsy, the examination of the death scene and the revision of the clinical history (Hunt, 2001).

According to Hannah and collaborators (Kinney & Thach, 2009) there exists no consensus about how SIDS should be defined. For instance, the definition of SIDS found in Medline reads as follows: the sudden, unexplained death of an infant younger than one year old. Some people call SIDS "crib death" because many babies who die of SIDS are found in their cribs (MedlinePlus, 2011). The National Institute of Health consensus conference issued the first standardized definition of sudden infant death in 1969 and defined it as the 'sudden death of an infant or young child, which is unexpected by history, and in which a thorough post mortem examination fails to demonstrate an adequate cause of death. The definition required thus an autopsy for all infants, who died from a similar condition as SIDS to establish a set of infants showing similar characteristics for whom vital statistics, research, and family counseling were needed' (Hannah et al., 2009). Furthermore, the authors stated that 'although SIDS was defined as a syndrome, and thus potentially the result of more than one disease, many observers still viewed SIDS as a single entity, because of its distinctive features, which included a peak incidence at 2 to 4 months of age, male predominance, and the presence of intrathoracic petechiae. Subsequent modifications of the definitions of SIDS restricted the application of the diagnosis, SIDS, to infants under the age of 12 months, added the requirement of a death-scene investigation, or linked the death to a sleep period (i.e., the time when the majority of deaths occurred). It is still unclear whether SIDS occurs during sleep or during the many transitions between sleep and arousal that occur during the night, since such deaths are typically not witnessed'. It has to be noted that heterogeneity of the definitions of SIDS has lead to contradictory results in scientific studies (Kinney & Thach, 2009).

The incidence of SIDS in industrialized countries ranges between the lower taxes found in Japan (0.09 cases per 1000 infants) to the higher taxes found in New Zealand (0.80cases per 1000 infants); United States has an intermediate rate (0.57 cases per 1000 infants) (Moon et al. 2007).

Epidemiological studies have identified several risk factors for SIDS, which are mainly related to pregnancy and postnatal period. Among these risk factors, mother's tobacco consumption represents one of the most important preventable causes of SIDS. For instance, if one third of the mothers smoked during and after pregnancy, 25 % of all cases of SIDS might be attributable to this (Carrion & Pellicer, 2002).

A quantitative systematic revision has found that infant, who suffered SIDS were two times more exposed to passive smoking than those who were not (OR=2.08 and 1.94 for prenatal and postnatal maternal tobacco consumption, respectively). There is evidence showing that there is a higher postnatal exposition to ETS, when both parents smoke during pregnancy (Anderson & Cook, 1997).

A recent ecological study conducted from 1995 to 2006 has shown that for every 1% absolute increase in the prevalence of smoke-free households with children, the rates of SIDS decrease by 0.4% (Behm et al., 2011.

2.2 Respiratory symptoms and illness

Several studies have shown an increased frequency of common respiratory symptoms of children (cough, sputums and wheezes) when parental smoking was present (US Surgeon General, 2006; Cook & Strachan, 1999) . A meta-analysis conducted by Samet and Sockrider revealed that parental smoking was associated with respiratory symptoms (asthma, wheeze, cough, rise of sputums or dyspnea of their children (OR ranged between 1.23 and 1.35). The highest risks were found when both parents smoked (see Table 1) (US Surgeon General, 2006).

2.2.1 Infections of the lower respiratory tract

During the first years of life of children, increases in respiratory problems of children are related to parental smoking habits. If both parents smoke the presence of wheezes and asthma increases by 20%. At the same time, infections of the lower respiratory tract and cough increases by 30% and by 13%, respectively (Zmirou et al. , 1990). These circumstances are directly related to the consumption of tobacco by the mother. For instance, bronchial infection with wheezes are 14% more frequent when mothers smoke more than 4 cigarettes per day, and 49% more frequent when they smoke more than 14 cigarettes per day (Neuspiel et al., 1989).

	Either parent smokes			One parent smokes			Both parents smoke		
	N	OR	95%CI	N	OR	95%CI	N	OR	95%CI
Asthma	31	1.23	(1.14-1.33)	7	1.01	(0.84-1.22)	10	1.42	(1.30-1.56)
Wheeze *	45	1.26	(1.20-1.33)	13	1.18	(1.10-1.26)	14	1.41	(1.23-1.63)
Cough	39	1.35	(1.27-1.43)	18	1.27	(1.14-1.41)	18	1.64	(1.48-1.81)
Phlegm △	10	1.35	(1.30-1.41)	7	1.24	(1.10-1.39)	6	1.42	(1.19-1.70)
Breathlessness △	6	1.31	(1.14-1.50)						

N: Number of studies
* Excluding EC study, in which the pooled odds ratio (OR) was 1.20
△ Data for phlegm and breathlessness restricted as several comparisons are based on fewer than five studies.
Adapted from USDHHS 2006, The Surgeon General's Report and Jonathan M Samet, Marianna Sockrider, Secondhand smoke exposure: Effects in children (Available at: www.uptodate.com, last accessed 19th October 2011)

Table 1. Effects for respiratory symptoms in children whose parents smoke according to the meta-analysis conducted by Samet and Sockrider

Bronchiolitis usually takes place among the first six months of life. Children with bronchiolitis history tend to present more bronchial spasms during early years and asthma among adolescence. This is why bronchiolitis is often considered as a risk factor that precedes repeated crisis of bronchial spasms and wheezes until the age of eight. Subsequently, passive smoking constitutes a risk factor for the appearance for asthma symptoms in infancy (Martin et al., 2003). Moreover, several studies have found that after the implementation of more restrictive tobacco law, hospitalizations of infants due to asthma decreased by 18.2% (Carriazo & Cuevo, 2010; Mackay et al., 2010).

Recently, a systematic revision including a meta-analysis has been published. The objective of this study was to explore if family tobacco consumption is related to low respiratory tract infections (LRTI) in children. This meta-analysis included more than 60 studies and showed that, if the father smokes, the OR for LRTI is 1.22 (95%CI: 1.10-1.35), if both parents smoke, the OR for LRTI is 1.62 (95%CI: 1.38-1.89) and that if any other member of the family also smokes, the OR for LRTI rises up to 1.62 (95%CI: 1.45-1.73). The strongest association of passive smoking with bronchiolitis was found when any other member of the family, besides the parents, also smoked (OR: 2.51; 95%CI: 1.96-3.21). Consequently, the authors concluded that passive smoking of cohabitants in children's households is the most important risk factor for LRTI. This risk is especially high, if the mother smokes during the postnatal period (Jones et al., 2011).

In some studies LRTI has been related to maternal tobacco consumption, but several oriental countries, as for example China and Vietnam, where maternal tobacco consumption is not frequent, show that paternal tobacco consumption itself can explain the rise of the incidence of LRTI (Jones et al., 2011; Suzuki et al., 2009; Chen et al., 1986).

Certain studies have shown that the effect of passive smoking of babies on respiratory illnesses is critical during the first year of life, since this is the period when the baby stays more time with his or her parents, even though important effects of passive smoking on respiratory illnesses have been found during school age (Oberg et al., 2011).

2.2.2 Asthma

The etiology of asthma is yet not clearly established. Some authors have related asthma to a higher frequency of respiratory infections in early life or to other inflammatory mechanisms of the pulmonary epithelium (Boulay & Boulet, 2003).

Several published scientific revisions have shown that there is a clear relationship between the prevalence and severity of asthma and the exposition to tobacco smoke in early life (US Surgeon General, 2006; Cook & Strachan, 1999).

Some authors speculate that smoking during pregnancy can alter pulmonary development in utero, which can be related to a higher risk for the development of asthma later in life (Milner et al., 1999). Other authors consider that SHS might be closely related to an allergic sensitization, however not a clear a clear association between tobacco smoke exposure and allergy has been established (Cook & Strachan, 1999).

There is clear epidemiologic evidence for an association of exposition to SHS with the risk to suffer asthma in childhood (US Surgeon General, 2006; Goksor et al., 2007). Table 1 shows the excess risk when parents or only the mother smokes. Although there is a dose response relationship between SHS and asthma, a well defined safety threshold level without risk has not been established (Institute of Medicine, 2007). Surgeon General's Report in 2006 revealed a relationship between the prevalence of SHS and asthma, but not with the incidence of asthma (US Surgeon General, 2006). Moreover, the exposure to tobacco smoke during early years is associated with a higher prevalence of asthma in adults (Larsson et al., 2001; Svanes et al., 2004).

Finally, numerous studies have related the tobacco smoke exposure to different clinical outcomes such as an increase in a) number of visits to the emergency departments due to asthma, b) clinical symptoms, c) number of medicines and d) other clinical parameters (Carlsen & Lodrup, 2005).

2.2.3 Other respiratory illnesses

Altet and collaborators found a positive association between passive smoking in infancy and a higher risk to develop pulmonary tuberculosis (Altet et al., 1996).

2.3 Middle ear illnesses

Some studies have suggested an association of parental smoking with the presence of middle ear illnesses in children. (Adair-Bischoff & Sauve, 1998; Kum-Nji et al. 2006). The meta-analysis conducted by the US Center of Disease Control and Prevention found a pooled odds ratio of 1.37 (95% CI 1.10-1.70) for recurrent middle ear otitis, 1.33 (95% CI 1.12-1.58) for middle ear effusions, and 1.20 (95% CI 0.90-1.60) for clinical referrals or operative interventions for middle ear effusions, if either parent smoked (US surgeon General, 2006).

Another meta-analysis concluded that middle ear illnesses were associated to prenatal smoking (OR:1.1), postnatal smoking (OR:1.46) and paternal smoking (OR: 1.27), the association is even higher if cohabitants, apart from the parents, smoke at home (OR: 1.35) (Royal College of Physicians, 2010).

2.4 Meningitis

A recently published article shows a significant positive association between passive smoking with invasive meningococcal bacteriological illness, as well as an increased carriage of *N. meningitides* and *S. pneuomoniae* (Lee et al., 2010). Another recent scientific revision revealed that parental smoking (one or both parents) doubled child's risk to suffer a meningitis (OR: 2.30; 95%CI: 1.74-3.06) (Tobacco Advisory Group, 2010).

2.5 Dental caries

A possible effect of second hand smoke on the development of dental caries in children is not clearly established; a recently published scientific revision has failed to demonstrate a potential association of second hand smoke with caries, maybe due to the heterogeneity of the studies included (Hanioka et al., 2011).

3. Strategies to reduce passive smoking in babies

There are four main strategies to try to reduce exposure to passive smoking of babies: education, regulation, legislation and litigation (Davis, 1998). These strategies mainly depend on administrative measures. Nevertheless, the role of health professionals concerning the education of their patients is critical, in order to protect non-smokers from passive smoking and promote smoke-free spaces (Samet & Sockrider, 2011).

The role of pediatricians and especially pediatrics residents is of vital importance as concluded in a study published in 2008 (Hymowitz et al., 2008). The study evaluated the efficacy of a special program for training pediatric residents to address tobacco and reduce exposure to tobacco smoke. As stated by authors 'The percent of parents who smoke at sites associated with the special training condition, but not of those at sites associated with standard training, who reported that residents advised them to stop smoking, offered to help them quit, and provided quit smoking materials increased significantly from baseline to year 4'.

The above listed strategies should also focus on women in reproductive age and on pregnant women, since both conditions are the two first exposure patterns of exposure to tobacco among babies. Different types of interventions have been developed and applied to promote smoking quitting during pregnancy and in the maternal-child environment (Jane et al., 2006; Salleras et al., 2003).

The emergence of health protection laws has addressed limitations of tobacco use in public. Closed spaces for smokers have been proved to be useful measures to prevent respiratory diseases in workers. For instance, the Spanish law 42/2010 prohibits the exposure of babies to tobacco smoke in public, closed places. However it does not regulate the exposure in private areas such as in the car or at home. Hence, a pediatric program in Primary Care should be defined and promoted, including interventions among families to reduce the exposure to SHS in children. In Spain pediatricians regularly follow up children's health status, and they would be the most appropriate professional group to promote passive smoke protection among children (Altet et al., 2007; Ortega et al., 2010).

In order to reduce infant exposure to ETS in private spaces, it is necessary to encourage parental (or baby sitters) smoking cessation. If not possible, smoke-free households could be promoted as well as the avoidance of smoking in the presence of a baby.

In Spain, the above mentioned law increases the awareness of smokers about the convenience of smoking in open-air spaces to protect others at work and public places; consequently parents, who smoke are more predisposed to adopt strategies to protect their children and other family members (see Appendix 2).

According to the last national survey of health (2006), the prevalence of adult smokers in Spain is 26.44% (21.51% in women and 31.56 in men) (see Appendix 3); in young adults the prevalence ascends up to 35 %, in spite of the fact that in the last years the number of smokers generally has decreased. Nonetheless, the number of babies exposed to tobacco smoke is still considerable (INE, 2006). Consequently, the reduction of the prevalence of smoking individuals (mainly the parents or the baby sitters) continues to be the most effective way to reduce exposure to passive smoking among infants. The following policies have contributed substantially in the reduction of the prevalence of smokers: a) increment of policies to control tobacco consumption, b) increased tobacco taxes, c) promotion of awareness about tobacco related health problems by informative advertisement, campaigns, and d) the increase of sanitary protection devices to help smokers in their cessation (Tobacco advisory Group, 2010). Programs directed to reduce the prevalence of smokers are those measures that mainly contribute to achieve smoke-free domiciles (Thomson et al., 2006).

4. Theories of change

In the previous chapter, we review the strategies to reduce ETS exposure in children. However, ultimately, reduce the exposure of children depends on parents and / or caregivers. Therefore, in this section, we review the theoretical foundations and implementation, based on some articles that determines the effectiveness of interventions to reduce children's exposure to passive smoking, and how has been carried out by parents. It is a systematic review of 2008 (Priest, N.), which included 36 studies. Sixteen of 36 them expressly employed a theoretical framework in the design and/or development of the intervention.

In 1994 McIntosh developed the activities for the parent manual based on behavior modification theory. Groner 2000 employed the health belief model, and Wakefield 2002 used a harm minimization approach. Abdullah 2005 based counseling strategies on the stages of change component of Prochaska's transtheorical model. Krieger 2005 was also guided by the trastheorical stages of change model, as well as by social cognitive theory.

The Motivational Interviewing, was used by Emmons 2001, Curry 2003 and Chan 2005. Chan 2006a used Ajzen's theory of planned behavior in the development of their educational intervention.

Greenberg 1994, Elder 1996, Conway 2004 and Fossum 2004 employed the social learning model.

Now, in this section we will review the most important theories concerning modifications of behavioral patterns will be presented. We have divided them in three levels following the ecological perspective of the scientific revision made by Glanz and collaborators in 1997 (Glanz et al., 1997).

CONCEPT	DEFINITION
Intrapersonal level	Individual characteristics that influence behavior, such as knowledge, attitudes, beliefs, and personality traits
Interpersonal level	Interpersonal processes and primary groups, including family, friends, and peers that provide social identity, support, and role definition
Community level	
Institutional factors	Rules, regulations, policies, and informal structures, which may constrain or promote recommended behaviors
Community factors	Social networks and norms, or standards, which exist as formal or informal among individuals, groups, and organizations
Public policy	Local, state and federal policies and laws that regulate or support healthy actions and practices for disease prevention, early detection, control and management

Note: Table published by Glanz et al. 1997

Table 2. An ecological perspective: Levels of influence

4.1 Individual or Intrapersonal level

The Health belief model by Janz and Becker (Janz & Becker, 1984) proposes that when someone deems it best to change a behavioral pattern, both advantages and disadvantages of this change are taken in consideration, followed by a rational decision. In addition, the perception of the individual susceptibility to the problem that requires a behavioral change and the severity of the problem are both taken into account. Recently, the concept of auto-efficiency has been added to this model. Auto-efficiency, a concept originally taken from Bandura's work (Bandura, 2011), defines an individual's confidence in undertaking a specific change in conduct.

The Health action model by Tones (Tones, 1991) is based on the previous model, but incorporates also the concept of self-esteem. Self-esteem is defined in this model as the individual's beliefs on his or hers qualities, and how they are perceived by others. Furthermore, this model includes a number of factors, such as previous knowledge and environmental features that can influence decision-making in the process of individual behavioral change.

The Theory of Reasoned Action / Planned Behavior by Ajzen (Ajzen, 1991) characterizes conduct depending on behavioral intention, subjective regulations and attitudes. This model specifies that real behavior is predicted by someone's intention to realize a

behavior. Hence, intention is the result of attitudes and subjective rules. Ajzen later modified and included the concept of "perceived behavioral control" that reflects, how easy or difficult an individual can perceive the task to follow a certain behavioral pattern.

The Transtheoretical Model was proposed by Prochaska y DiClemente (Prochaska & DiClemente, 1983). This model describes the phases in conduct change, and is one of the newest models describing behavioral change. It is also known as 'transtheoretical model' since it incorporates the structures of other, older models. This model considers behavioral change as a dynamic process –instead of a static process-, which takes into account the fact that, rapidity for behavior change is different in each individual and that changes occur in time following five stages. This stages are: 1) precontemplative: the individual does not think about possible behavioral changes; 2) contemplative: the individual is thinking about a change; 3) preparation: the individual enters a necessary path to be able to perform a conduct change; 4) action: the individual carries out the change in a short period of time; and 5) maintenance: the individual maintains a behavioral change over a period of time, (usually measured as keeping the change for at least six months). The transtheoretical model includes the possibility of relapses in earlier phases. This means that a maintained behavior change can also be achieved after a cyclical process of progresses and relapses. This model has been broadly used, but continues to be controversially discussed (Katz, 2001; Littlell et al., 2002; van Sluijs et al., 2004; Whitelaw et al., 2000).

The Precaution Adoption Process Model proposed by Weinstein (Weinstein, 1988), This model includes seven phases: not being informed or aware of a problem (unprepared), without interest in the problem, deciding about intervention, determined not to act, acting and maintenance. These phases represent qualitative models of different behavioral patterns, beliefs and experiences, and the factors influencing the transitions between the different phases can vary. Weinstein believes that this model is linear, and that interventions require being adapted to each phase of the model. It displays similarities to the transtherorical model of behavioral change.

4.2 Interpersonal level

Social learning theory or social cognitive theory of Bandura (Bandura, 2001) postulates that people learn by observing someone else's behavior and apply it to themselves. Both, the credibility and reinforcement of the learned conduct are fundamental. This theory goes beyond individual factors influencing behavioral changes. It includes environmental and social factors. The key elements of this theory are summarize in table 3 (Cooper, 2000; Redding et al., 2000). The self-efficacy has been evaluated as an important predictor of the success in the proposed behavioral change (Cheng, 1999).

Differential Association-Reinforcement Theory (Glanz et al., 1997) is based on the circumstance that we can adopt new behavioral patterns by looking and imitating other persons. There are positive and negative reinforcements (price and punishment, for example). It mainly takes into account what happened after conduct change. Behavioral patterns are imitated leading to different levels of reinforcement, taking into account exposure and consequences of the conduct.

Theory	Focus	Key Concepts
Health Belief Model	Considers the pros and cons for behaviour change, as well as the perception, susceptibility and severity of the illnesses	Perceived susceptibility Perceived severity Perception of benefits from action Action barriers Auto-efficiency
Health Action Model	To promote people's self-esteem. To find environment support	Self-esteem Own beliefs Knowledgements Favourable environment
Transtheoretical Model	The intention to change varies among individuals and in time periods. The relapse is a normal phase in the process of change	Precontemplation Contemplation Preparation Action Manteinance Relapse
The Precaution Adoption Process Model	Changes need of certain phases and intervention should be adapted to those phases.	Without information Without interest Deciding what to do Decided to act Decided not to act Acting Manteinance
Social Learning Theory or Social Cognitive Theory	Considers the credibility of social models. Positive reinforcement. Helps conductal maintenance	Environment Situation Conductal capacity Expectation Hope Self-control Observational learning Reinforcements Self-efficacy Emotional aspects Reciprocal determinism
Differential Association-Reinforcement Theory	We learn new behavioural patterns by looking at and imitating others and by positive and negative reinforcements. The subject defines a behavioural pattern as good or justified according to his or her commitment. It takes into account what happens once a conduct change initiated.	Imitation Positive reinforcements Negative reinforcements Consequences of the behaviour
Self-Regulation Theory	Behaviour is defined by the interaction between subject and environment. Self-efficacy is a key concept as well as the personal standards.	Interaction environment-subject Self-efficacy Personal standards
Harm reduction model	Necessity to reduce health risks related to drug consumption, at both individual and community level.	Respect Acceptance Support Promotion of own's capacities (empowerment)

Table 3. Summary of the theories of change

4.3 Community level

Self-Regulation Theory (Baumeister et al., 2004). Behavior is seen as the sum of interactions between the individual and environment. Self-efficacy is the key question. Response is related to our personal values. It has been studied in the following fields: exercise, stress, alimentary behavior, cardiovascular disease and drug consumption.

Harm reduction model developed, among others, by Newcombe and O'Hare (Newcombe et al., 1995) is based on the principles of respect, acceptance, support and promotion of the own capacities (empowerment). This model was generated as an answer to the accumulating evidence of serious health risks related to alcohol overconsumption and tobacco use. Later on, it has been used for the understanding of behavioral pattern changes related to the consumption of drugs and to HIV infection. The model aims to diminish the negative effects of drug consumption, and does not imply quitting completely the drug consumption (O'Hare et al., 1995).

Some authors (Nigg et al., 2002), postulate that these theories can help us to elucidate, why a person is motivated to initiate a behavioral change. Other authors, in contrast, emphasize more on the reasons, why a certain conduct is being hold in time. They also suggest that for different health problems, different models can be useful, which at different stages of behavioral change can explain better these changes. Finally, multiple interventions concerning a series of health related problems (for instance, obesity and tobacco use or alcohol consumption) may need inputs from several theories at different phases or stages, to be able to explain in an improved way behavioral patterns (Martin, 2006).

5. Conclusions

There is enough scientific evidence to conclude that indirect tobacco smoke exposure of children (and adults) has negative health effects. Tobacco smoke exposure of children can cause: low tract respiratory infections, middle ear infections, asthma, low weight at birth and sudden death syndrome.

Subsequently, strategies to reduce passive exposure to tobacco are an urgent and priority sanitary, public health aim. Scientific evidence should enforce actions performed by health care professionals of all disciplines to undertake measures in order to eradicate this avoidable risk in children.

6. Key points

- Environmental tobacco smoke is made from the smoke exhaled by smokers and the smoke produced during the combustion of cigarettes.
- Passive smoking is the leading cause of preventable death in infancy in industrialized countries and one of the first leading causes of the rise of cancer in developing countries.
- Up to 70 % of the western children live in households where at least one of the parents smokes. Thirty percent of these children are exposed every day to tobacco smoke.
- Sudden infant death syndrome, acute respiratory illnesses, acute and chronic middle ear infections and meningitis are related to ETS.

-   Passive smoking during pregnancy lowers baby's weight at birth, highers the risk of: prematurity, congenital malformations, spontaneous abortion and fetal and perinatal mortality.
-   The rise of the policies controlling tobacco consumption, the increase in of tobacco taxes, the awareness of tobacco related health problem in advertising informative campaigns, and the increase of sanitary devices to help smokers in their cessation have contributed to reduce the number of smokers.
-   Reducing the prevalence of smokers among parents and baby sitters continues to be the most effective way to prevent passive smoking among children.

Compound	Does it cause cancer?
Nicotine	
Dimethylnitrosamine	
Benzopyrene	X
Pyrene	X
Napthalene	X
Phenol	
Acetone	X
Methanol	
Vinyl	
Carbon Monoxide	X
Nitrogen oxides gases	
Tolue	
Benzene	
Arsenic	
Cadmium	X
Niquel	
Lead	
Naphthylamine	X
Toluidine	X
Polonium-210	X
Ammonia	
Dibenzocridine	X
Cianamide	
DDT	
Uretane	
Butane	

Adapted from: Departament de Salut de la Generalitat de Catalunya (http://www.gencat.cat/salut/depsalut/pdf/gtabacp.pdf, last accessed November 10th 2011) and Cancer Society of New Zeland Inc. and Health Promotion Services Branch Health Dept. of Western Australia

Appendix 1. Main components of tobacco smoke and its carcinogenic effect

Exposure	Does NOT avoid exposure	Avoids exposure
At home	To smoke at home when the bay is not there	Not smoking at home, in any room
	To smoke in delimitated areas of the house	Prohibit family members and visitators to smoke in the house
	To smoke with the window or balcony open	To always smoke outside the house. To smoke only in the balcony or terrace keeping the door closed
	To smoke and ventilate the house after smoking	
In the car	To smoke in the car when the bay is not there	Not to smoke in the car, even though the baby is not there
	To smoke in the car when the baby is there but with the window opened	

From: Ortega G, Castellà C, Martín-Cantera C, Ballvé JL, Díaz E, Saez M, et al. Passive smoking in babies: the BIBE study (Brief Intervention in babies. Effectiveness). BMC Public Health. 2010;10:772.

Appendix 2. Measures to avoid exposure to tobacco smoke in babies

	Number	%
Men		
Total	5,794.60	31.56
16-24 years old	596.3	24.96
25-34 years old	1,580.90	40.16
35-44 years old	1,382.40	37.41
45-54 years old	1,141.30	38.83
55-64 years old	654.2	28.45
65-74 years old	312.4	18.64
≥75 years old	127	8.93
Women		
Total	4,101.70	21.51
16-24 years old	657	28.93
25-34 years old	1,108.40	30.16
35-44 years old	1,093.00	30.73
45-54 years old	845.6	28.47
55-64 years old	286.5	11.77
65-74 years old	83.9	3.86
≥75 years old	27.3	1.37

From: Spanish Ministry of Health. National Health survey, 2006

Appendix 3. Tobacco consumption in Spain. Daily number of smokers (in thousands) and percentage aged ≥ 16 according to sex and age group

7. Abbreviations

CI: Confidence Interval
CO: Carbon monoxide
ETS: Environmental Tobacco Smoke
IARC: International Agency for the Research on Cancer
LRTI: Low respiratory tract infections
OR: Odds Ratio
SHS: Second Hand Smoke
SIDS: Sudden Infant Death Syndrome
WHO: World Health Organization

8. References

Abdullah ASM, Lam TH, Mak YW, Loke AY. A randomizes control trial of a smoking cessation intervention parents of young children: a randomised controlled trial. Addiction 2005: 100(11): 1731-40.

Adair-Bischoff CE, Sauve RS. Environmental tobacco smoke and middle ear disease in preschool-age children. Arch Pediatr Adolesc Med 1998 Feb;152(2):127-33.

Altet MN, Alcaide J, Plans P, Taberner JL, Salto E, Folguera LI, et al. Passive smoking and risk of pulmonary tuberculosis in children immediately following infection. A case-control study. Tuber Lung Dis 1996 Dec;77(6):537-44.

Altet N, Pascual MT, Grupo de Trabajo sobre Tabaquismo en la Infancia. Tabaquismo en la infancia y adolescencia. Papel del pediatra en su prevención y control. An Esp Pediatr 2007;52:168-77.

Ajzen I. The theory of planned behavior. Organizational Behavior and Human Decision Processes 1991;50:179-211.

Anderson HR, Cook DG. Passive smoking and sudden infant death syndrome: review of the epidemiological evidence. Thorax 1997 Nov;52(11):1003-9.

Bandura A. Social cognitive theory: an agentic perspective. Annu Rev Psychol 2001;52:1-26.

Baumeister F, Vohs K. Handbook of Self-Regulation. Research, Theory, and Applications . Edited by Roy F Baumeister and Kathleen D Vohs 2004.

Behm I, Kabir Z, Connolly GN, Alpert HR. Increasing prevalence of smoke-free homes and decreasing rates of sudden infant death syndrome in the United States: an ecological association study. Tob Control 2011 Apr 7.

Boulay ME, Boulet LP. The relationships between atopy, rhinitis and asthma: pathophysiological considerations. Curr Opin Allergy Clin Immunol 2003 Feb;3(1):51-5.

Carlsen KH, Lodrup Carlsen KC. Parental smoking and childhood asthma: clinical implications. Treat Respir Med 2005;4(5):337-46.

Carriazo N, Cuervo J. Universalizar los espacios sin humo parece disminuir los ingresos hospitalarios en niños. Evid Pediatria 2010;6:84.

Carrion F, Pellicer C. El tabaquismo pasivo en la infancia. Nuevas evidencias. Prevencion del Tabaquismo 2002;4(1):20-5.

Chan SS, Lam TH, Salili F, Leung GM, Wong DC, Botelho RJ, et al. A randomized controlled trial of an individualized motivational intervention on smoking cessation for parents of sick children: a pilot study. Applied Nursing Research 2005;18(3):178-81.

Chan SS, Lam TH. Preventing exposure to second.hand smoke. Seminars in Oncology Nursing 2003;19(4): 284-90

Chen Y, Li W, Yu S. Influence of passive smoking on admissions for respiratory illness in early childhood. Br Med J (Clin Res Ed) 1986 Aug 2;293(6542):303-6.

Cheng TL, DeWitt TG, Savageau JA, O'Connor KG. Determinants of counseling in primary care pediatric practice: physician attitudes about time, money, and health issues. Arch Pediatr Adolesc Med 1999 Jun;153(6):629-35.

Conway TL, Woodruff SI, Edwards CC, Hovell MF, Klein J. Intervention to reduce environmental tobacco smoke exposure in Latino children: null effects on hair biomarkers and parents reports. Tobacco Control 2004; 13(1): 90-2.

Cook DG, Strachan DP. Health effects of passive smoking-10: Summary of effects of parental smoking on the respiratory health of children and implications for research. Thorax 1999 Apr;54(4):357-66.

Cooper MD. Towards a model of safety culture. Safety Science 2000;36(2):111-36.

Curry SJ, Lundman EJ, Graham E, Stout J, Grothaus L, Lozano P. Pediatric-based smoking cessation intervention for low-income women: a randomized trial. Archives of Pediatrics and Adolescent Medicine 2003;157(3):295-302

Davis RM. Exposure to environmental tobacco smoke: identifying and protecting those at risk. JAMA 1998 Dec 9;280(22):1947-9.

Doll R, Hill AB. Smoking and carcinoma of the lung; preliminary report. Br Med J 1950 Sep 30;2(4682):739-48.

Elder JP, Perry CL, Stone EJ, Johnson CC, Yang M, Edmundson EW, et al. Tobacco use mesurement, prediction, and intervention in elementary schools in four states: the CATCH Study. Preventive Medicine 1996;25(4):486-94.

Emmons KM, Wong M, Hammond SK, Velicer WF, Fava JL, Monroe AD et al. Intervention and policy issues related to children's exposure to environmental tobacco smoke. Preventive Medicine 2001:32:321-31.

Environment and Health Information System (ENHIS). Exposure of children to second-hand tobacco smoke. fact sheet 3 4 December 2009; (Available in ttp://www.euro.who.int).

Fossum B, Arborelius E, Bremberg S. Evaluation of a counseling method for the prevention of childe exposure to tobacco smoke: an example of client.centered communication. Preventive Medicine 2004;38(3): 295-301.

Glanz K, Rimer BK. Theory at a Glance. A Guide for Health Promotion Practice. National Cancer Institute, National Institutes of Health, U S 1997;Washington, DC., Department of Health and Human Services. NIH Pub. 97-3896.

Goksor E, Amark M, Alm B, Gustafsson PM, Wennergren G. The impact of pre- and post-natal smoke exposure on future asthma and bronchial hyper-responsiveness. Acta Paediatr 2007 Jul;96(7):1030-5.

Greenber RA, Strecher VJ, Bauman KE, Boat BW, et al. Evaluation of a home-based intervention program to reduce infant passive smoking and lower respiratory illnes. Journal of Behavioral medicine 1994;17(3):273-90.

Groner JA, Ahijevych K, Grossman LK, Rich LN. The impact of a brief intervention on maternal smoking bejavious, Pediatrics 2000;105(1 Pt 3): 267-71.

Hanioka T, Ojima M, Tanaka K, Yamamoto M. Does secondhand smoke affect the development of dental caries in children? A systematic review. Int J Environ Res Public Health 2011 May;8(5):1503-19.

Harlap S, Davies AM. Infant admissions to hospital and maternal smoking. Lancet 1974 Mar 30;1(7857):529-32.

Hymowitz et al. The pediatric residency training on tobacco project: four-year parent outcome findings. Prev. Med. 2008, Aug;47(2):221-4. Epub 2008 Jun 30.

Hunt CE. Sudden infant death syndrome and other causes of infant mortality: diagnosis, mechanisms, and risk for recurrence in siblings. Am J Respir Crit Care Med 2001 Aug 1;164(3):346-57.

IARC. Tobacco Smoke and Involuntary Smoking. Vol. 28. Lyon. IARC Monographs 2002.

Institute of Medicine. Exposure to environmental tobacco smoke. In: Clearing the Air: Asthma and Indoor Air Exposures National Academy Press, Washington DC 2000;278.

Instituto Nacional de Estadística. Encuesta Nacional de Salud de España. Ministerio de Sanidad y Consumo 2006.

Jane M, Martinez C, Altet N. Guia clínica per promoure l'abandonament del consum de tabac durant l'embarás. Departament de Salut 2006.

Janz NK, Becker MH. The Health Belief Model: a decade later. Health Educ Q 1984;11(1):1-47.

Jones LL, Hashim A, McKeever T, Cook DG, Britton J, Leonardi-Bee J. Parental and household smoking and the increased risk of bronchitis, bronchiolitis and other lower respiratory infections in infancy: systematic review and meta-analysis. Respir Res 2011;12:5.

Katz DL. Behavior modification in primary care: the pressure system model. Prev Med 2001 Jan;32(1):66-72.

Kinney HC, Thach BT. The sudden infant death syndrome. N Engl J Med 2009 Aug 20;361(8):795-805.

King K, Martynenko M, Bergman MH, Liu YH, Winickoff JP, Weitzman M. Family composition and children's exposure to adult smokers in their homes. Pediatrics 2009 Apr;123(4):e559-e564.

Krieger JK, Takaro TK, Allen C, Song L, Weaver M, Chai S, et al. The Seattle-Kong Country healthy homes project: implementation of a comprehensive approach to improving indoor environmental quality for low-income children with asthma. Environmental Health perspectives 2002;110 Suppl 2: 311-22

Kum-Nji P, Meloy L, Herrod HG. Environmental tobacco smoke exposure: prevalence and mechanisms of causation of infections in children. Pediatrics 2006 May;117(5):1745-54.

Larsson ML, Frisk M, Hallstrom J, Kiviloog J, Lundback B. Environmental tobacco smoke exposure during childhood is associated with increased prevalence of asthma in adults. Chest 2001 Sep;120(3):711-7.

Lee CC, Middaugh NA, Howie SRC, Ezzati M. Association of Secondhand Smoke Exposure with Pediatric Invasive Bacterial Disease and Bacterial Carriage: A Systematic Review and Meta-analysis. PLoS Med 2010 Dec 7;7(12):e1000374.

Littell JH, Girvin H. Stages of change. A critique. Behav Modif 2002 Apr;26(2):223-73.

Lopez MJ, Perez-Rios M, Schiaffino A, Nebot M, Montes A, Ariza C, et al. Mortality attributable to passive smoking in Spain, 2002. Tob Control 2007 Dec;16(6):373-7.

Mackay D, Haw S, Ayres JG, Fischbacher C, Pell JP. Smoke-free legislation and hospitalizations for childhood asthma. N Engl J Med 2010 Sep 16;363(12):1139-45.

Martin C. La factibilidad del consejo preventivo sobre accidentes de tráfico en atención primaria. Tesis Doctoral Universidad Autonoma de Barcelona 2006.

Martin C, Roig L, Ferrer S, Jane C, Vilella E. Los niños y su exposición al tabaquismo pasivo. 3er Congreso del CNPT. Zaragoza. 2003. Ref Type: Personal Communication.

McIntosh NA, Clark NM, Howatt WF. Reducing tobacco smoke in the environment of child with asthma: a cotinine-assisted, minimal-contact intervention. Journal of Asthma 1994;31(6): 453-62.

MedlinePlus. Available at: http://www.nlm.nih.gov/medlineplus/

Milner AD, Marsh MJ, Ingram DM, Fox GF, Susiva C. Effects of smoking in pregnancy on neonatal lung function. Arch Dis Child Fetal Neonatal Ed 1999 Jan;80(1):F8-14.

Moon RY, Horne RS, Hauck FR. Sudden infant death syndrome. Lancet 2007 Nov 3;370(9598):1578-87.

Neuspiel DR, Rush D, Butler NR, Golding J, Bijur PE, Kurzon M. Parental smoking and post-infancy wheezing in children: a prospective cohort study. Am J Public Health 1989 Feb;79(2):168-71.

Newcombe R, O'Hare PA, Matthews A, Buning EC. The reduction of drug-related harm. A conceptual framework for theory, practice and research 1992; London; Routledge.

Nigg CR, Allegrante JP, Ory M. Theory-comparison and multiple-behavior research: common themes advancing health behavior research. Health Educ Res 2002 Oct 1;17(5):670-9.

Oberg M, Jaakkola MS, Woodward A, Peruga A, Pruss-Ustun A. Worldwide burden of disease from exposure to second-hand smoke: a retrospective analysis of data from 192 countries. Lancet 2011 Jan 8;377(9760):139-46.

O'Hare PA, Newcombe A, Matthews EC, Buning ED. La reducción de los daños relacionados con las drogas. Barcelona, Grup Igia 1995;17-39.

Ortega G, Castella C, Martin-Cantera C, Ballve JL, Diaz E, Saez M, et al. Passive smoking in babies: the BIBE study (Brief Intervention in babies. Effectiveness). BMC Public Health 2010;10:772.

Priest N, Roseby R, Waters E. et al. Family and carer smoking control programmes for reducing children's exposure to environmental tobacco smoke (Review). The Cochrane Database Syst Rev. 2008, Oct 8; (4):CD001746.

Prochaska JO, DiClemente CC. Stages and processes of self-change of smoking: toward an integrative model of change. J Consult Clin Psychol 1983 Jun;51(3):390-5.

Redding C, Rossi J, Rossi S, Velicer W, Prochaska JO. Health Behavior Models. The International Electronic Journal of Health Education 2000;3(Special Issue):180-93.

Roseby R, Waters E, Polnay A, Campbell R, Webster P, Spencer N. Family and carer smoking control programmes for reducing children's exposure to environmental tobacco smoke. Cochrane Database Syst Rev 2003;(3):CD001746.

Royal College of Physicians. Passive smoking and children. A report by the Tobacco Advisory Group London: RCP, 2010.

Salleras L, et alt. Guia per a la prevenció i el control del tabaquisme des de l'àmbit pediàtric. Departament de Sanitat i seguretat social Generalitat de Catalunya 2003.

Samet J, Sockrider M. Secondhand smoke exposure: Effects in children. UpToDate 2011.

Samet J, Sockrider M. Control of secondhand smoke exposure. UpToDate 2011; ttp://www.uptodate.com/.

Seong MW, Moon JS, Hwang JH, Ryu HJ, Kang SJ, Kong SY, et al. Preschool children and their mothers are more exposed to paternal smoking at home than school children and their mothers. Clin Chim Acta 2010 Jan;411(1-2):72-6.

Suzuki M, Thiem VD, Yanai H, Matsubayashi T, Yoshida LM, Tho LH, et al. Association of environmental tobacco smoking exposure with an increased risk of hospital admissions for pneumonia in children under 5 years of age in Vietnam. Thorax 2009 Jun;64(6):484-9.

Svanes C, Omenaas E, Jarvis D, Chinn S, Gulsvik A, Burney P. Parental smoking in childhood and adult obstructive lung disease: results from the European Community Respiratory Health Survey. Thorax 2004 Apr;59(4):295-302.

Thomson G, Wilson N, Howden-Chapman P. Population level policy options for increasing the prevalence of smokefree homes. J Epidemiol Community Health 2006 Apr;60(4):298-304.

Tobacco Advisory Group. Passive smoking and children. Royal College of Physicians 2010.

Tones K. Health promotion, self empowerment and the concept of control. Leeds Polytechnic, Leeds 1991.

US Surgeon General. The Health Consequences of Involuntary Exposure to Tobacco Smoke: A Report of the Surgeon General.U.S. Dept. of Health and Human Services, Centers for Disease Control and Prevention, Coordinating Center for Health Promotion, National Center for Chronic Disease Prevention and Health Promotion. Office on Smoking and Health, Atlanta, Georgia 2006.

US Surgeon General. Reducing the health consequences of smoking: 25 years of progress. US Department of Health and Human Services 1989;DHHS publication No (CDC) 89-8411.

van Sluijs EMF, van Poppel MNM, van Mechelen W. Stage-based lifestyle interventions in primary care - Are they effective? American Journal of Preventive Medicine 2004;26(4):330-43.

Wakefield M, Banham D, McCaul K, Martin J, Ruffin R, Badcock N, et al. Effect of feedback regarding urinary cotinine and brief tailored advice on home smoking restrictions among low-income parents of children with asthma: a controlled trial. Preventive Medicine 2002;34(1):58-65.

Weinstein ND. The precaution adoption process. Health Psychol 1988;7(4):355-86.

Whitelaw S, Baldwin S, Bunton R, Flynn D. The status of evidence and outcomes in Stages of Change research. Health Educ Res 2000 Dec;15(6):707-18.

Zmirou D, Blatier JF, Andre E, Ferley JP, Balducci F, Rossum F, et al. [Passive smoking respiratory risk. A quantitative synthesis of the literature]. Rev Mal Respir 1990;7(4):361-71.

Permissions

The contributors of this book come from diverse backgrounds, making this book a truly international effort. This book will bring forth new frontiers with its revolutionizing research information and detailed analysis of the nascent developments around the world.

We would like to thank Oreste Capelli, for lending his expertise to make the book truly unique. He has played a crucial role in the development of this book. Without his invaluable contribution this book wouldn't have been possible. He has made vital efforts to compile up to date information on the varied aspects of this subject to make this book a valuable addition to the collection of many professionals and students.

This book was conceptualized with the vision of imparting up-to-date information and advanced data in this field. To ensure the same, a matchless editorial board was set up. Every individual on the board went through rigorous rounds of assessment to prove their worth. After which they invested a large part of their time researching and compiling the most relevant data for our readers. Conferences and sessions were held from time to time between the editorial board and the contributing authors to present the data in the most comprehensible form. The editorial team has worked tirelessly to provide valuable and valid information to help people across the globe.

Every chapter published in this book has been scrutinized by our experts. Their significance has been extensively debated. The topics covered herein carry significant findings which will fuel the growth of the discipline. They may even be implemented as practical applications or may be referred to as a beginning point for another development. Chapters in this book were first published by InTech; hereby published with permission under the Creative Commons Attribution License or equivalent.

The editorial board has been involved in producing this book since its inception. They have spent rigorous hours researching and exploring the diverse topics which have resulted in the successful publishing of this book. They have passed on their knowledge of decades through this book. To expedite this challenging task, the publisher supported the team at every step. A small team of assistant editors was also appointed to further simplify the editing procedure and attain best results for the readers.

Our editorial team has been hand-picked from every corner of the world. Their multi-ethnicity adds dynamic inputs to the discussions which result in innovative outcomes. These outcomes are then further discussed with the researchers and contributors who give their valuable feedback and opinion regarding the same. The feedback is then collaborated with the researches and they are edited in a comprehensive manner to aid the understanding of the subject.

Apart from the editorial board, the designing team has also invested a significant amount of their time in understanding the subject and creating the most relevant covers. They scrutinized every image to scout for the most suitable representation of the subject and create an appropriate cover for the book.

The publishing team has been involved in this book since its early stages. They were actively engaged in every process, be it collecting the data, connecting with the contributors or procuring relevant information. The team has been an ardent support to the editorial, designing and production team. Their endless efforts to recruit the best for this project, has resulted in the accomplishment of this book. They are a veteran in the field of academics and their pool of knowledge is as vast as their experience in printing. Their expertise and guidance has proved useful at every step. Their uncompromising quality standards have made this book an exceptional effort. Their encouragement from time to time has been an inspiration for everyone.

The publisher and the editorial board hope that this book will prove to be a valuable piece of knowledge for researchers, students, practitioners and scholars across the globe.

List of Contributors

L. Cegolon
Padua University, Department of Molecular Medicine, Padua, Italy

L. Cegolon and G. Mastrangelo
Imperial College London, School of Public Health, S. Mary's Campus, London, UK

J. H. Lange
Envirosafe Training and Consultants, Pittsburgh, Pennsylvania, USA

Namrata Kotwani, Ruqayyah Abdul-Karim and Marion Danis
Department of Bioethics, National Institutes of Health, USA

James F. Cawley
Department of Prevention and Community Health, USA

Roderick S. Hooker
School of Public Health and Health Services, USA

Diana Crowley
School of Medicine and Health Sciences, The George Washington University, USA

Giancarlo Lucchetti, Alessandra L. Granero Lucchetti, Rodrigo M. Bassi1, Alejandro Victor Daniel Vera and Mario F. P. Peres
São Paulo Medical Spiritist Association, Brazil

Giancarlo Lucchetti
João Evangelista Hospital, Brazil

Giancarlo Lucchetti, Alejandro Victor Daniel Vera and Mario F. P. Peres
Federal University of São Paulo, Brazil

Alaneir de Fátima dos Santos, Humberto José Alves, Cláudio de Souza, Simone Ferreira dos Santos, Rosália Morais Torres and Maria do Carmo Barros de Melo
Telehealth Center, School of Medicine, Federal University of Minas Gerais, Brasil

Jumana Antoun
American University of Beirut, Lebanon

Oreste Capelli, Imma Cacciapuoti and Antonio Brambilla
The District Primary Care, Emilia-Romagna Region, Bologna, Italy

Silvia Riccomi and Marina Scarpa
General Practitioner, Dept of Primary Care, Modena, Italy

Nicola Magrini
Drug Evaluation Unit, Emilia-Romagna Health Agency, Bologna, Italy

Elisabetta Rovatti
Dept of Pneumology – University Hospital – University of Modena and Reggio Emilia, Italy

Caroline da Rosa
Fundação de Atendimento Sócio-Educativo do Rio Grande do Sul (FASE/RS), Brazil

Jose María Arribas Blanco and María Hernández Tejero
Faculty of Medicine, Autonomous University of Madrid, Madrid, Spain

Lourdes Rofes Ponce
Drug Dependency Unit at Sant Joan de Reus Hospital, Reus, Spain

Ricardo Almon
Family Medicine Research Centre School of Health and Medical Sciences, Örebro University, Örebro, Sweden

Elisa Puigdomènec
Lifestyles Research Group from the Primary Health Care Research Unit of Barcelona, IDIAP Jordi Gol, Barcelona, Spain

Manuel A Gomez-Marcos
Department of Medicine, University of Salamanca, Cardiovascular Research Group (RETICS RD06/0018/0027, REDIAPP), Carlos III Institute of Health of the Spanish Ministry of Health, SACYL, Primary Care Research Unit, La Alamedilla Health Center, Salamanca, Spain

Carlos Martín-Cantera
Lifestyles Research Group from the Primary Health Care Research Unit of Barcelona, IDIAP Jordi Gol, Lifestyles Research Group (RETICS RD06/0018/0027, REDIAPP), Carlos III Institute of Health of the Spanish Ministry of Health, Department of Medicine, University Autonomus of Barcelona, Passeig de Sant Joan Health Center, Barcelona, Spain